Lost and Found

The Misadventures of a Reluctant Trekker

Donna Abel

Donna Abel

Copyright © 2025 Donna Abel

All rights reserved. No part of this book may be reproduced, distributed, or transmitted in any form or by any means, including photocopying, recording, or other electronic or mechanical methods, without the prior written permission of the author, except in the case of brief quotations used in critical reviews and certain other non-commercial uses permitted by copyright law.

This is a work of creative nonfiction. While based on actual events, some names, characters, and incidents have been fictionalised for narrative purposes. Any resemblance to actual persons, living or dead, is purely coincidental.

For permissions or inquiries, contact:
innkedin.com/in/donnaabel

First published in 2025
ISBN: 978-1-0369-2677-9

Cover design by Anna Anderson
Printed in UK, USA

Dedication

In memory of my mother.

This story might be a bit raw, honest, and unfiltered, maybe more than you expect, but that's what makes it real, and she would have loved it.

Acknowledgements

To all of my family and friends who gave me the confidence to write this and the inspiration to complete it. Your belief in me has made this possible. Thank you to those who have agreed to have their names included in the book.

To the past, current, and future residents of Jersey Cheshire Home, who provide such inspiration to those of us who have the good fortune to trek on their behalf. I hope this book raises awareness of the amazing work carried out by all staff and volunteers at the home – a charity that is making a real and meaningful difference.

Some elements of this book echo events in my own life. I'll leave it to you, dear reader, to decide which sections draw on reality and which are purely fiction.

Introduction

Hi. I'm Samantha. And I am *not* a trekker.

Well ... not a natural one, anyway.

Yet, what started as a smug charity auction victory (with wine in hand and ego in overdrive) soon spiralled into early-morning hikes, a life lived almost exclusively in waterproofs, and an unforgettable poop-related incident that I'll probably never live down. And that was all before the trek had even begun.

After losing my mum, navigating grief, burnout, and what may or may not have been the onset of menopause, I needed a radical change. Needed to laugh again. Needed purpose. Needed to move, physically and emotionally. And the best place to do that, apparently, was Vietnam.

What you'll find here is not a hiking how-to guide. It's a messy, sometimes mad, often TMI (too much information) story of what happens when a control freak with her own personal Karen – the name of my internal monologue – tries to rediscover herself ... one ridiculous step at a time.

There are moments of heartbreak. Moments of hilarity. And more than a few reminders that sometimes you need to get completely lost before you can learn who the hell you really are.

Plus, you're in the right place if you've ever

- overthought a swimsuit situation
- questioned your sanity mid-step
- tried to walk off grief
- shouted "Feck off!" to your own Karen
- or wondered what would happen if "the one who got away" suddenly made an unexpected reappearance in your life

The full, unexpurgated details are in my journal at the end of the book. First, though, I asked my good friend Donna to write an account of the year in which I became a bona fide trekker. I hope you enjoy the journey.

Lace up and let's get going.

Chapter 1

The Poolside Rivalry

Samantha felt a pang of irritation as she stood at the edge of the pool, staring at thirty-eight unoccupied sun loungers. With so many other options, why did that bloody woman have to place a towel on the lounger right next to hers?

Fifteen minutes in, she had completed thirty lengths and felt pretty good. Her breaststroke was improving, and her potentially slipped disc was holding up. Then she realized that her lounger neighbour was coming up to lap her for the fourth time. *Four times!* And she wasn't even swimming. She was walking along the bottom of the pool. Samantha's self-esteem hit the tiles.

As an only child, Samantha knew that she could be, let's say, passionately competitive. Even at three, she'd been determined to win at everything. She was inconsolable for hours after losing a game of pass the parcel. So being outpaced by a human crab was utter torture.

Her dad, Denis, had always admired what he called her drive. He loved how she turned every failure into fuel, seeing it as one of her greatest strengths, along with her sharp wit, her empathy, even her obstinacy.

But *this*? Being lapped every four minutes? This was spiritual warfare.

With the woman's towel still obnoxiously close, and small talk in swimsuits too awkward to bear, Samantha kept swimming. But she was swallowing more water with every lap. She should have tied her hair higher. Karen – Samantha's internal critic, the suburban queen of unsolicited complaints, inappropriate thoughts, and perfectly timed passive-aggressive heckles – was in rare form today, and the perpetual onslaught was tugging her down.

She lost track of the lengths. Was it thirty-four? Forty-four? Feck it. Let's call it thirty-eight. That felt about right. She decided to count down from twelve to zero. That would give her fifty in total … maybe.

She tried walking a length herself, but knew she looked like she'd been stung by a jellyfish. She laughed, and immediately inhaled more water. Who knew swimming could double as a hydration challenge?

***

The next day, Samantha checked the forecast. No rain. Fantastic. She could squeeze in a decent walk before work.

There was no more time to waste. She'd signed up for an arduous charity trek, and she needed to put in the hard yards. A gentle swim in the health-club pool simply wouldn't cut it.

Up at 5:15 a.m. and guess what?

It was bloody pissing down.

Typical.

Nevertheless, she managed three miles, dried off, pulled herself together, and stayed positive. For all its irritations, last night's swim had left her feeling sprightly. This morning's 8,700 steps felt good, too. She planned to increase the distance over the coming weeks, assuming she didn't catch pneumonia from her wet leggings first.

For a brief moment, she wondered why she was training in cold rain when Vietnam would be hot and humid. Perhaps she should do laps of a sauna instead? But hey, maybe a bit of suffering now would make it a breeze later.

"Planning, practice, and preparation make for high performance," she reminded herself.

"Better tell the Olympic Committee to reserve a space on the team," said Karen.

**

She completed three more solid walks, each exceeding 10,000 steps, over the next few days and suffered only a couple of blisters. But this week wasn't just about physical fitness.

She had to get her mind into shape, too.

Unfortunately, Karen was not exactly supportive. "You need a shrink, not a feckin' trek," she scoffed. "Mental fitness? What a joke. More like mental obesity."

Today marked three months since the sudden and heartbreaking passing of Samantha's beautiful mum. She had died on holiday, while making a cup of tea. It was a massive, devastating shock for the whole family. Samantha took some comfort from knowing that she hadn't suffered, but the loss was still unbearable.

They had been carbon copies of each other, and not just in appearance. They also shared the same spirit, charm, and wit ... and they were both as stubborn as hell. Her mum had been her rock. Her advisor. Her biggest fan. Losing her felt like losing a limb.

A heavy knot had lodged itself in Samantha's chest, just like the one she'd carried when her dad had passed eight years earlier. She found herself welling up at the smallest things: an ad on the telly, the sight of a favourite trinket, a smell that reminded her of home. But she pushed those feelings down. There was work to do.

She'd learned from her dad's passing that humour could be her shield. When Denis died, he left her a letter, a treasure, and a gift: the financial means to start her own consultancy. He had even registered the business years earlier, calling it SOS

Management Consultancy. Samantha O'Sullivan – her name, her future.

His belief in her meant everything.

She poured herself into the business with grit and determination. And it thrived.

Now, with the trek training underway, she knew thorough preparation was key: more protein, fewer carbs, sensible portions. She understood the theory, and was doing her best to put it into practice.

Home-cooked meals? Check.

Increase the step count each week? Check.

So, why was she gaining weight?

Cue a mental image of Bridget Jones and a soundtrack of mortifying, snack-related rationalizations.

Of course, Karen was straight in there, twisting the knife into the open wound. "Let's be honest, you're eating your feelings and everything else you can find. You're a human trash can. It's hardly surprising you're getting fatter. *Much* fatter. At this rate, you'll need a seatbelt extension for the flight to Vietnam. And DVT is a real possibility. You need to get a grip."

The voice was growing louder and more vindictive. They were now fighting on a daily basis. Samantha was still winning – her scorecard read eight rounds to four – but the gap was narrowing all the time.

Chapter 2

Menopause or Madness?

Samantha prided herself on being in control – of her business, her health, even her coffee order. So the seemingly inexorable rise in her weight was becoming a cause of concern. Summoning as much tact as she could manage, she asked her work colleagues for tips on how to shift the extra pounds.

"No eating between meals," said Rachel.

Samantha's face flushed at the thought of all those flapjacks, handfuls of nuts, and chocolate bars that were her "rewards" for completing each day's exercise.

"What about yoga? The hot one's great," suggested Sai.

"And there's that new injection," said Michael.

Rachel shot him a look that screamed, "For the love of God, shut the hell up!"

"Not that you need it," stammered Michael. "In fact, you probably wouldn't even qualify for it yet. Because … you know … you need to be *really* fat."

"*Jaysus* ... keep digging," said Sai, under her breath.

Karen couldn't control herself. "I told you it was getting out of hand. People are offering you advice on weight-loss injections. How's that for a wake-up call?"

Everyone got back to work, and Samantha consoled herself with a surreptitious brownie as she stood by the printer.

One of the account managers, Mary, who hadn't said a word during the earlier discussion, sidled over and whispered, "Samantha, darling, it's not the snacks. I've got one word for you – menopause."

Samantha blinked in disbelief. Surely that was a problem for much, *much* later. What the actual feck?

Karen jumped in immediately. "The cheek of her. That's ageist. You should fire her!"

But as a highly suggestible hypochondriac with a PhD in overthinking, Samantha was already wondering if Mary might be on to something. The comment didn't just land but dug in and started gnawing away at her, like a tick.

***

After three weeks of frantic Googling and fretting over worst-case scenarios, she finally caved and booked an appointment with her GP.

Unfortunately, Dr Heart was probably the most misnamed physician in the world. She had all the warmth of a tax audit, and her patience was wearing perilously thin after a number of previous health scares:

- Eyeball cancer? Nope – hay fever.
- Mouth cancer? Nope – use a softer toothbrush and start flossing.
- Brain tumour? Nope – get your eyes checked, you probably need reading glasses.

Samantha dreaded seeing her, especially after the incident. In what she now realized was a deeply misguided attempt to lighten the mood, she'd turned up for her smear test with a vajazzle.

Dr Heart's response had been a withering "Was that really necessary?"

Samantha had never wanted to evaporate more.

But she needed answers, so she was back in the consulting room, waiting for Dr Heart to look up from her notes. After what seemed like an eternity, the GP finally sighed and asked, "Okay, Samantha. What is it now?"

"I think I might be experiencing … symptoms."

"*Symptoms?* Of what?"

"Menopause."

Dr Heart chuckled, dryly. "Samantha. You're thirty-two."

"It can happen early."

"That's true. But let's stick to facts, rather than Google. Have you missed any periods?"

"No."

"Hot flushes?"

"No. But I've had cold sweats … occasionally … when I sleep. If I can ever get to sleep, that is."

"Let me ask you this. Have you spotted glitter in unusual places? Gem stones? Anything else sparkling when it shouldn't?"

"No," snapped Samantha. For feck's sake, it was one vajazzle. Can't she just let it go?

Dr Heart closed her file. "Let me guess. Someone put this idea in your head a couple of weeks ago and you've been spiralling ever since?"

"I've not been spiralling."

Silence.

"Fine. Maybe I have. A bit. But I can't ask my mum for advice any more, can I?"

Samantha could have sworn she detected a flash of sympathy, but it quickly vanished. The GP handed her a blood test slip. "Get this done. And for God's sake, stop consulting Dr Google."

"If I am in menopause, you'll owe me an apology."

"If you are, I'll bake you a cake."

"Lemon drizzle."

"Noted." Then, with surprising tenderness, the GP added, "How have you been doing since your mum passed? You mentioned not sleeping. Do you want to talk about it?"

What was going on? Why was Dr Heartless suddenly being so … kind?

"I'm fine."

"Okay. If you're sure. But remember I'm here. Or I can refer you if you'd rather talk to someone else."

Karen had been unusually taciturn throughout the consultation, but she couldn't hold her tongue any longer. "Give the woman a diploma. She's finally realized you need a shrink."

Samantha merely muttered, "Noted."

***

The following week, she organized a workshop titled: "Menopause Matters @ SOS: Does It Matter to You?" It was mandatory for the whole staff.

Afterwards, Mary approached her and leaned in close to whisper, "I'm so glad you've decided to face this head on."

Karen couldn't help herself. "What a bitch. Why didn't you fire her when you had the chance? She still thinks you're fifteen years older than you are. Maybe it's time to invest in some Botox."

Samantha just smiled sweetly and said, "Yes, we all need to understand what our colleagues are going through, even though it'll be years before some of us have to deal with it ourselves."

Chapter 3

The Lousy Dosser

Samantha was a notorious workaholic – single by choice, married to her work, and thriving in her self-built empire. Her late father's faith in her had lit a fire, and she was determined to keep it burning.

So, why was she a few weeks away from abandoning the consultancy, flying to Southeast Asia, and embarking on a charity trek?

The reason was pure, unfiltered rivalry.

It all started at a dinner dance to raise funds for Jersey Cheshire Home. She spotted her nemesis the instant she walked through the door.

Lorena Dean. One-time mentee turned business backstabber.

"What the actual feck is she doing here?" Samantha muttered to herself.

Karen added, "Bottom feeder alert. I bet she's here to poach another contract. She's shameless. Why not go and say hello and accidentally spill a glass of red wine on that dress of hers?"

Samantha knew she had to resist the temptation, though. There were nine important clients on her table, and they would be expecting a fun, relaxing night. So, despite Lorena's presence – unwelcome as a flat prosecco – she focused on remaining cool and playing the perfect host.

For the first couple of hours, everything went according to plan, with plenty of laughter, dancing … and drinking.

Then the MC announced the start of the main event of the evening – the charity auction. Several of Samantha's guests joined in the bidding, with the others cheering them on whenever they went way over their limit to win a lot. She herself stayed well out of it, though. Her donation had been made months earlier, when she'd booked the table.

After forty minutes of increasingly raucous bidding, the auctioneer eventually arrived at the final lot. "Now, ladies and gentlemen, we have something truly special," he announced with a flourish of his gavel. "A ten-day adventure through the beautiful countryside, mountains, and jungle of Vietnam. It's the perfect opportunity for anyone looking for a challenge. And remember, you'll be supporting a wonderful local charity that provides invaluable assistance to people living with physical disabilities. You'll be trekking to help those who can't. Who will start the bidding?"

Samantha's heart skipped a beat. She hadn't even realized she wanted it until her hand was in the air.

A trek through Vietnam. A test of endurance that would force her to push herself beyond her usual boundaries. And a chance to make a real difference in the lives of people whose own boundaries had been so cruelly restricted. She could feel the competitive fire rising up inside her. She was going to win this. She *had* to win this.

After a swig of champagne to steel herself, she called out, "One thousand pounds." Her voice echoed around the room as every head turned to face her.

Barely a second elapsed before another bidder shouted, "One thousand five hundred."

This time it was Samantha who turned, but she didn't need to. She already knew the identity of her rival. The voice was as smooth and taunting as ever. The smile perfect, polished, supercilious.

Samantha felt her jaw tighten, but she refused to be rattled. This was a game of strategy, a contest of wills, and she had to remain calm.

She and Lorena went back and forth, each outbidding the other. The price climbed higher and higher, but Samantha was resolute. She simply could not let Lorena win.

"Two thousand," she cried.

"Two thousand five hundred," Lorena shot back.

"Three thousand!"

The rest of the room had fallen silent, the atmosphere charged with electric tension. Everyone knew that this was getting out of hand, but no one dared to intervene. It was clearly personal.

Lorena, having been nurtured under Samantha's wing at SOS, had subsequently gone rogue. She'd left to start her own firm, LD Consultants (how original!), and immediately undercut SOS on a key project.

Hence the nickname – the Lousy Dosser.

This wasn't about the money for Samantha. It was about pride. About proving that, despite everything, she was still at the top of her game. Still the best.

Lorena raised her hand again. "Three thousand five hundred," she said, her eyes never leaving Samantha's.

"Four thousand," countered Samantha, laser focused, more determined than ever to deny the Lousy Dosser her moment of glory.

Lorena didn't hesitate. "Four thousand five hundred."

Samantha's mind raced. She had to change the pattern. Throw Lorena off her game. Gathering all the composure she could muster, she said, "Five and a half thousand."

Lorena's face fell as she reluctantly lowered her arm.

Victory!

Samantha punched the air in triumph, forgetting that every eye in the place was still on her. Then she started chanting: "Winner, winner, chicken dinner!"

Who cared what people thought, though? She had bested the Lousy Dosser.

***

It was a couple of hours later that reality started to dawn. Five and a half grand was a lot, but she could afford it. The real issue was the amount of time she'd have to devote to preparing for the trip.

"Oh God, what have I done?" she groaned.

She knew there'd be no half measures. Total commitment was in her DNA. Back in primary school, her class had been set the task of making tea cosies for the town's elderly residents. She'd knocked on doors, taken measurements of every teapot, and custom-made twenty cosies, each of which fitted perfectly.

Overachiever wasn't just her lane; it was her highway.

She'd launched her first consultancy straight after university, pouring everything she had into it. Then she'd watched it unravel and collapse. At first, she couldn't understand why established companies didn't want a twenty-one-year-old with no experience telling them what to do, but eventually the penny dropped.

Her solution was to work even harder on the next venture. That meant there was no time for love, so she missed her chance with Kev – the one who got away. It had all been worth it, though, to ensure a decent return on her dad's investment. Or so she'd always told herself.

Lately, she wasn't so sure. She enjoyed all the trappings of success, yet life had started to feel predictable, maybe even stale. It was time for a change. A new challenge.

"It'll be great," she told herself. "Get me out of my comfort zone."

"Or push you over the edge," said Karen.

Chapter 4
Finding the Perfect Partner

Despite her tough, self-reliant image – and boundless reserves of grit and determination – Samantha had never been too proud to ask for help when she needed it. And the monotony of her early-morning walking regime soon led to the realization that she needed it now … in the form of a training partner. Someone quietly supportive. Discreet.

Of course, she could have signed up with one of the thousands of personal trainers, fitness coaches, and wellness gurus who advertised their services online. But while she'd always been a generous donor to charity, she was as tight as a duck's arse when it came to spending money on herself. The thought of actually paying someone simply to walk alongside her made her skin crawl. And so the hunt for a volunteer began.

Memories of *Take Me Out*, *Blind Date*, and even one or two choice excerpts from *Naked Attraction* kept popping into Samantha's mind as she giddily started the process of locating her perfect walking partner. Her first port of call was LinkedIn.

Treating it like a recruitment process in which the most important qualification was a love of trekking, she eventually narrowed it down to two candidates.

"Both men, I see," said Karen. "What a surprise. There's only ever room for one princess in your relationships."

"Feck off," Samantha muttered aloud, stabbing at her scrambled eggs with unnecessary force. "You're wrong. I'm not a princess. I'm just a lonely, potentially peri-menopausal woman who needs some help. And anyway, what do you know? You don't even exist!"

For once, there was no comeback, so she turned her attention to the list of requirements she'd compiled the night before:

Essential

1. Strong legs, shoulders, back, and glutes
2. A good sense of humour and kindness
3. Time for training and lots of patience
4. Exceptional listener and a person of few – but funny – words

Preferable

1. Speaks English and sweats minimally
2. Smells good even when sweating, and is happy to help
3. Punctual, enjoys walking, willing to share food

> 4. First-aider, GP, or paramedic with a comprehensive first-aid kit

Samantha studied the list with all the intensity of a detective who was struggling to solve a cold case. "Have I missed anything?" Then it hit her. "Oh my God. Of course. How could I forget that?"

It went in the "Essential" column:

> 5. Absolutely no connection – or resemblance – to the Lousy Dosser in any way, shape, or form.

Then she underlined it and added an arrow pointing to the top of the list to indicate it was actually the number-one requirement – just above a fully functioning body.

There was nothing to indicate that either of the LinkedIn candidates knew Lorena. And their macho profile pictures certainly suggested they'd be fit enough to keep pace with Samantha on the training walks. But then she started to think that Karen may have had a point. Why had she narrowed it down to two men? She was looking for a walking partner, not a husband.

She closed the laptop and decided to try a different approach.

"Good for you," said Karen. "Although there's nothing stopping you looking for both at the same time. You're already in your thirties. At this rate, you're destined to die alone, with a chin full of whiskers, surrounded by seven cats."

"Fine by me," replied Samantha. "Maybe I'll name them after the Seven Dwarfs."

With that, she picked up her phone and Googled the local paper's classified section. A chatbox appeared and invited her to key in her ad. She typed:

LOOKING TO HAVE SOME FUN? EARLY-MORNING EXERCISE WITH NO STRINGS. ATTACHED. PLEASE CONTACT KATIE GREEN

She reasoned you couldn't be too careful. This sort of thing was a magnet for weirdos. There was no way she'd ever give them her real name at this stage.

Next, she had to provide an email address, so she hastily created one for Katie.

Finally, she clicked the "All Platforms" option for maximum exposure, and indicated she wanted the ad to run for three days. The whole thing cost £1.60. What a bargain! "Let's see," said Karen.

Chapter 5

The Lowdown

Although it was now several weeks since the auction, Samantha realized she still had absolutely no idea what a charity trek actually entailed. So she arranged a meeting with the charity's CEO to get the lowdown on precisely what she'd signed up for.

First, though, she sought a little advice from her old friend Dr Google ... or, in this case, Trekker Google. The search "How to prepare for a trek in Vietnam" yielded the following results:

1. Research Your Destination. Look into specific trekking spots like Sapa, Ha Giang, or Pu Luong. Check difficulty levels, terrain, weather conditions, and whether permits are needed.
2. Plan Your Itinerary. Be realistic. Choose a route that matches your fitness level. Map out start/end points, trails, and accommodation.
3. Pack Essentials. Sturdy backpack, hiking boots, layers, rain jacket, hat, sunglasses, sunscreen,

first-aid kit, headlamp, water bottle, snacks, and maybe a light sleeping bag.
4. Get Vaccinated. Ask your GP about required vaccinations (typhoid, hepatitis A and B, tetanus).
5. Build Fitness. Trekking is demanding. Start walking, jogging, or cycling to improve stamina and leg strength.
6. Consider Hiring Local Guides. Especially useful for tougher trails. Guides = knowledge + safety.
7. Respect Local Culture. Remain mindful and kind, and practise sustainable tourism.

Samantha sat back in her chair, her heart racing. "What on earth have I done?" she sighed. "Maybe it's not too late to drop out."

"Get vaccinated?" screamed Karen. "For a walk? I warned you. This might kill you. And as for stamina. Strength. Well, you're fecked on both counts. Better just quit now before you make an even bigger fool of yourself."

Samantha instinctively put her hands over her ears, even though she knew the voice was inside her head. She didn't want to hear it. She wanted–no, she *needed* an adventure.

***

From the very start of the meeting, it was clear that Eloise – the CEO of Jersey Cheshire Home – was not one for pulling her punches.

"You're lucky with this one," she said. "You're not camping, and there's usually running water in the homestays. But don't expect any bathrooms along the route. If you need to go, find a bush."

Jesus, Mary, and Holy St. Joseph, thought Samantha, trying not to flinch. *What is this? A charity walk or corporal punishment?* Hoping to steer the conversation in a more encouraging direction, she asked, "Do you think I'll lose much weight?"

Eloise laughed. "God, no. If anything, you'll gain a few pounds." Sensing it wasn't the answer Samantha had hoped for, she added, "But they'll be good pounds. By the time you've finished, you'll be fitter than you've ever been in your life."

Was that a dig? Samantha suddenly felt defensive. "I've been walking every morning since the auction."

"Well done," said Eloise. "How many miles?"

"I'm up to four," said Samantha, proudly.

"You'll need to increase that to fifteen to twenty miles a day, through tough terrain and at elevation."

Samantha replied with a casual nod and scribbled something in her notepad, as if she'd just received confirmation of her own training schedule, but the thought filled her with dread. How on earth was she meant to walk just short of a marathon every morning?

Eloise smiled. "Don't worry. It's fifteen months to the trek, so you've got plenty of time to build up your stamina. But you'd better start now if you want to enjoy it. Otherwise, it won't be much fun when you arrive in Vietnam. I'll be organizing some group walks over the winter. They act like a mutual support system, and they're a great way to connect with your fellow-trekkers before you start sharing rooms."

Sharing rooms? Samantha nearly choked on her coffee. *I could have booked a private apartment in the Bahamas for less than this.*

"Punishment disguised as a charity. Perfect for you, Sammie," chortled Karen. "You can think of all the mojitos you're missing out on while you're having a crap in the jungle. Fantastic!"

Samantha asked who else had signed up, but Eloise explained that she couldn't share that information due to GDPR restrictions.

Seriously? thought Samantha. *Wasn't that designed to protect bank details, not the names of sweaty walkers?*

"I can tell you there'll be a couple of doctors on the trip. They'll keep everyone in check."

Samantha hoped neither of them was a psychiatrist. She didn't want anyone challenging her sudden fear of confined spaces if sharing a room got to be too much for her.

The meeting ended with Samantha assuring Eloise that she'd think about the group hikes. In truth, though, she'd already set her heart on a personal walking buddy – someone to keep her motivated without the pressure of enforced socializing.

It was time to check Katie Green's inbox.

Chapter 6

Warning: Flashing Images

Samantha's jaw dropped. She double-checked the address: KatieG*1992@gmail.com. Yes, that was the one she'd created and submitted to the paper. Yet somehow, in the space of four days, it had received 12,456 emails.

"Wow," she said. "People must really love walking."

Her excitement faded fast.

The first few messages made it painfully clear that her ad was open to quite liberal interpretations. She reread it slowly:

- Looking to have some fun?
- Early-morning exercise
- No strings attached

She burst out laughing. It was so outrageous, it was almost impressive. She scrolled through the inbox, morbidly curious to see if she recognized any of the names.

Unable to resist, she started replying to a few … especially those who had been kind enough to attach a picture:

- "Too small."

- "Weak glutes."
- "Have you no shame?"
- And her personal favourite: "I'd recommend seeing your GP. Urgently."

It was like a crash course in human anatomy – all shapes, sizes, and a host of unfortunate angles.

More than once, she shrieked, "Jaysus, I'll never be able to unsee that!"

But she ploughed her way through all 12,456 of them. She figured it was the least she could do after creating this mess.

Finally, though, she admitted defeat.

The Katie Green plan had backfired. Spectacularly.

Even if she did manage to find what seemed to be a pearl amongst the dirty swines, she knew there'd always be a little voice in her head asking, "Is this guy an early riser … or an early riser?"

"That's it," she muttered. "No more personals. No more LinkedIn roulette. Time to face the music."

She would have to bite the bullet and sign up for Eloise's group hikes.

There were sure to be some awkward conversations, but she could handle that. Some people she didn't get along with? Inevitably, but she'd dealt with them her whole life. It was only when she started thinking about their relative hiking experience that she really started to worry. Everyone else had probably been yomping across the hills for years, and there'd she be, in her brand-new boots, wondering if she was doing it right, but too scared to ask.

She found herself staring at people on the street, suddenly fascinated by their different gaits, shuffles, power walks, even the occasional limp. She noted one man striding ahead while his partner practically jogged to keep up. The whole dynamic was weirdly hypnotic.

She'd never realized walking was so complicated.

Curiosity got the better of her. She filmed herself walking in stilettos. (Fabulous, of course.) Then in her new hiking boots. (Train wreck: they turned her into a plodding duck with weak ankles.) But she could hardly trek through the jungle in her latest pair of Jimmy Choo's, so she designed three different walks in the boots, filming each one in turn. Then she sent the videos to her leadership team, pretending it was for a research project.

"Which walk seems most confident?" she asked.

Walk #2 won, but it involved awkward, long strides and a subtle shuffle.

Effective? Possibly.

Ridiculous? Certainly.

"Why not place another ad?" suggested Karen. "You could say, 'Hi, I'm Samantha.

You may know me as Katie, the author of a softcore dating ad that appeared in last week's paper. But I swear I just want a walking buddy.' I'm sure people will believe you."

There was nothing else for it. She'd just have to turn up at the group hike with her own natural, inefficient, unconfident walking style and hope that the rest of them didn't laugh her off the hillside.

Chapter 7

Becoming a Groupie

Eloise had thoughtfully provided Samantha with a list of essential outdoor clothing, so she would be properly equipped for the first hike. After plenty of research (and more than a little Pinterest doomscrolling), she finally found a brand she liked – Patagonia. They were committed to sustainability – offering lifetime repairs for all their products – top quality, and their colours really popped. Plus, their form-fitting trousers did wonders for her glutes.

She went wild with her credit card. Knickers, bra, socks, T-shirt, fleece, anorak, even her hat were all emblazoned with the Patagonia logo. She may not have been an experienced hiker, but she was determined to look like one.

"You muppet. Did Patagonia adopt you? You look like a walking billboard."

Samantha didn't care what Karen thought. For once, she felt brave. This was about trusting her gut, and her gut was telling her she looked like she could climb Everest.

"Right, Samantha," she said out loud. "It's time to meet the others and get walking."

***

"The others" turned out to be a small group of hikers of varying degrees of experience and ability, just as Eloise had promised. One stood out from the crowd, though. He had a calm, grounded energy, a cheeky smirk, and a slightly disconcerting habit of raising his eyebrows to emphasize a point, almost like punctuation marks.

He took a long, lingering look at Samantha as she strolled over, which made her wonder if he was admiring her new gear or the body inside it.

As shy and introverted as she could sometimes be, she was well aware that her tall, athletic physique and smooth, sun-kissed skin were like catnip to many men – especially outdoor types. And today her auburn hair, which was usually tied up in a practical bun, was falling in a gorgeous cascade across her shoulders.

Eyebrow-raising man flashed a sly smile as she approached the group, then casually stepped behind her.

Here we go, she thought. *I've barely got here and he's already making a move.*

Then she felt a couple of gentle tugs, first at the nape of her neck, then at her waist. She glanced over her shoulder and saw the man's hand holding two price tags. He grinned and handed them over.

Samantha was mortified.

Karen cackled. "Oh dear, Sammie. I guess there's no turning back. You can't return them now."

After recovering a little of her composure, Samantha sought out Eloise. "I've been practising my walk," she confided.

"Most people your age don't need to practise. But I'm looking forward to seeing it."

Once the walk had started, Samantha remained alongside Eloise in the middle of the pack, chatting comfortably. Eloise mentioned that they were on the hunt for another doctor for the Vietnam trek, as one of their regular GPs had unexpectedly pulled out.

"It's a real shame because Emily was perfect. No nonsense. Doesn't suffer fools. Always makes sure everyone finishes. It's so unlike her to drop out like this."

Samantha hesitated, then asked if there was anything she could do to help.

"Well," Eloise replied, "do you know any good GPs who might be prepared to volunteer?"

Samantha chuckled at the thought of Dr Heart striding through the jungle with a group of exhausted trekkers trailing in her wake. "I don't think you'd ever forgive me if I put you in touch with my doctor. She's cold, blunt, totally lacking in compassion. Ironically, her name's Dr Heart, but I call her Dr Heartless."

She glanced over at Eloise, expecting at least a smile, but at first all she saw was shock.

"Wow! You don't hold back, do you? Perhaps I should call you Sammie Savage." Then Eloise's face softened and creased into conspiratorial grin. "Your Dr Heartless is our Emily ... *and my sister-in-law*." She barely got the last word out before bursting into laughter.

"Oh my God, Eloise, I'm so sorry. I had no idea."

"It's fine, really," said Eloise, still giggling. "Actually, I appreciate the honesty. But for what it's worth, I do think she's a terrific doctor ... on a trek at least. Before her, we had to make do with Dr Pat. Sturdy woman. Powerful legs. Zero common sense. We were in Iceland. She went behind a rock for a call of nature. Unfortunately, the rock was at the top of a mountain, so she could be seen for miles around."

Samantha gasped.

"Oh, but it gets worse," Eloise spluttered, tears now streaming down her face. "She scooped up her business, popped it in a poo bag, tied it to her backpack, and marched proudly into town. It swung from side to side like some sort of bizarre trophy."

Samantha gagged. "That's vile."

"No one else could poo for the rest of the trek," Eloise wheezed. "So maybe now you'll understand why I'm hoping Emily has a change of heart. We don't want another Dr Pat."

"Five and a half grand, Sammie. Money well spent. Sound like you'll have a blast," said Karen.

Eloise went on to explain that she always shared the list of prospective trekkers with the doctors, just so they could check everyone was fit enough to participate. Two days later, Emily had withdrawn from the trip. When Eloise had pressed her for a reason, she'd blurted out that one of the group was a narcissistic hypochondriac who was likely to cause trouble.

Samantha swallowed hard. "Just button it, Karen," she muttered under her breath.

Chapter 8

An Unexpected Explosion

Samantha was starting to enjoy the group hikes. Especially this one. It was a crisp, dry, gusty autumn day, although the ground was still slick from what felt like weeks of relentless rain.

The group had decided on a daring route: the Southern Loop. Just over half a marathon in length, it promised around four hours of scenic challenge. They would traverse quiet country lanes, wind through the parishes of St Lawrence and Trinity, pass through Victoria Village, and descend toward Grand Vaux before returning to the heart of St Helier.

Samantha was in her element, soaking in the tranquillity. No tech, no contracts, no office politics, just nature, movement, and peace. Bliss.

They were heading towards the scheduled pit stop at the Orchid Museum. Tricia, one of the trekkers, was beyond relieved to spot it from the hilltop as she'd been bursting for a pee for over an hour. But the day took a dramatic turn as they started the descent.

Samantha took a tumble. Or rather a full-blown, spectacular wipeout. As she lost her footing, she reached out in desperation and grabbed hold of her neighbour Julie, who in turn grabbed Tricia. The three of them all went down in a chain reaction of flailing limbs, screaming as they landed with a thump in a tangled, soggy heap.

The shock of it all was too much for poor Tricia, who looked down forlornly at the wet patch that was forming on her trousers. It wasn't caused by the sodden ground. She staggered to her feet, red-faced with a slightly bruised tailbone, but it was her pride that had taken the biggest hit.

"You clumsy oaf. She'd have been fine if you'd managed to stay upright. Poor Tricia."

Samantha ignored Karen's rebuke and instead apologized profusely to Tricia and Julie, but soon all three of them were laughing again.

"I guess it'll make a good tale for the campfire," said Tricia with a shrug.

To anyone watching from a distance, it must have looked like an epic game of human dominoes. Despite the mishap, though, Samantha was finally starting to feel like she belonged. She was comfortable and relaxed with these people, and they seemed genuinely fond of her, too. She could hardly wait for the next hike.

But life had other plans for her.

Her work schedule suddenly went into overdrive, which meant the only time she could spare for training was first thing in the morning. However, the group hikes had taught her that it was much easier to clock up the miles with some company, so she returned to the tricky task of trying to recruit a walking buddy.

Of course, she was more than a little wary following the Katie Green debacle, but it surely couldn't hurt to post a message on the WhatsApp group that Eloise had set up for the Sunday hikers.

"I'm walking tomorrow morning from White Rock. If anyone fancies joining, I'll see you there. Leaving at 5:15 *sharp*!"

There were no replies, but that was hardly unusual for the group, so she still held out hope that someone – most likely Julie or Tricia – might show up.

She rolled out of bed at 4:45, brushed her teeth, splashed some cold water on her face, and pulled on her walking gear. She'd grown to love the White Rock walk, especially at dawn. The view of the sun climbing out of the ocean never got old.

She arrived at 5:05 and was intrigued to see a car already in the lay-by. A man in a black peaked cap was sitting inside. Playing it cool, she remained in her own car until 5:14, then jumped out, ready to go. To her surprise, the man stepped out too.

"Samantha?" he asked, walking towards her.

"Yes …" she replied, a slight edge of caution in her voice.

"I'm James. I'm on the charity trek to Vietnam."

Samantha stared at the face, then flushed as she realized who it was. Price-tag man! Her embarrassment over the incident had caused her to avoid him for the rest of that hike, and he hadn't turned up since. But now here he was, standing in front of her. And those familiar raised eyebrows suggested he remembered her, too. "Nice to meet you properly. Shall we get going?"

Samantha was pleasantly surprised to find that James was relatively normal, and that he seemed to tick most of the items on her list of walking buddy requirements. Moreover, he let her set the pace, which she appreciated. As they walked and talked, it soon became clear that James had quite a lot of trekking experience. As for training, he said he preferred early walks in small groups – get it done and dusted before the day began.

He was light-hearted and funny, didn't take himself too seriously, and, best of all, didn't ask her anything about her work, personal life, or bank balance. She returned the favour and didn't pry into his private life, either.

Then, without warning, he said, "You know, there was a random advert in the local paper a few weeks ago. Someone looking for a walking partner. I replied but never heard back."

Samantha blinked. "That's odd," she said, picking up the pace slightly.

Karen screeched, "I knew he was too good to be true! You've seen his bits! Do you remember what they looked like?"

Trying to remain calm, Samantha asked casually, "Really? What did the ad say?"

James shrugged. "I can't really remember. Aside from the fact that the woman who posted it – Katie, I think her name was – specified that she wanted to walk early in the morning. I felt a bit sorry for her. Probably some desperate housewife hoping to get a sunrise photo to liven up her Instagram story."

"*What?*" said Samantha sharply. "Why would you think that? Maybe she just didn't want to walk alone."

James seemed momentarily startled by her reaction. Up shot the eyebrows. "Either way," he said, "it was all a waste of time. I hate time-wasters, don't you?"

Samantha flashed a tight smile and quickly changed the subject. "Have you met many of the others who are going on the trek?"

"A few," James replied.

"*And ...*" she prompted.

"They all seem fine." He paused for a moment, seemingly weighing up whether he knew her well enough to continue. "With one exception. A woman called Loz ... Lola ...

something like that. I only met her once, but I found her a bit much. Her perfume nearly choked me. And as for her personality … I'd describe her as a self-important pampered princess."

"Really? Go on …" Samantha was curious.

"I'm no psychologist, but she struck me as a total narcissist. Kept boasting about the fact that she'd set up her own company. Who the hell cares? We're here to walk, not network with potential new clients. But hey, there's one on every trek. You just need to give them a wide berth." He shot Samantha a sideways glance and asked, "You're not a princess, are you?"

Samantha smirked. "No. But you're a real Prince Charming, aren't you?"

"Just thought I'd better check. I don't want to be stuck in the jungle with two of them. By the way, I've been called Prince Charming a few times before. But I prefer Lothario."

"*Lothario?*" Samantha raised her own eyebrows. "What does that even mean?"

"Darling," said James with a grin, "it's an idle man who spends his time surrounded by the rich and famous."

"Understood," said Samantha with a chuckle. "Thanks for the warning."

They maintained a good pace and finished slightly breathless, sweaty, and upbeat.

"So, should we make this a regular thing?" James asked as they reached their cars.

"Absolutely," Samanatha replied. "I'll be in touch."

On the drive home, her mind kept returning to him. He seemed like her kind of person, yet he'd been one of the respondents to Katie's ad. She had to know what he wrote – and if he attached any jpegs – but that would have to wait till the evening. For now, she barely had time to shower and change if she was going to make it into the office on time.

Chapter 9
Sleepless Nights and Poopy Pants

By the time she got home, exhausted after yet another soul-sucking day at SOS, Samantha didn't have the energy to scroll through 12,456 emails in search of the one from James. Instead, she climbed straight into bed and prayed for sleep.

But Karen was in no mood to let her rest.

"What if he's a mass murderer? Or a serial abuser? What if he's not even on the trek? He could have just stumbled across that group hike and joined in. No one really talked to him, did they? What if his name isn't even James, just like yours isn't Katie?"

The tossing and turning continued until 4:24 a.m., when Samantha finally admitted defeat. Karen had won. She grabbed her phone and scrolled through Katie's inbox for five minutes until she came across the name "James Ahern" in the sender column.

She held her breath and clicked on the message. It read:

Hi Katie

I'm taking part in a trek for charity next year. In the past, I've found it easier to walk with someone, as it helps me stay accountable and actually get out of bed to train, knowing I've got someone to meet.

I'm an excellent timekeeper, have some walking experience, and I'm even first-aid trained. Hope to hear from you soon.

All the best

James

No hint of sleaze. A reassuring reference to the charity trek. Nothing out of character for the man she'd walked with the previous morning. And, most importantly, no photo attachments!

Satisfied, Samantha rolled over and promptly fell asleep.

She awoke half an hour later in a puddle of sweat. Ah, the joys of peri-menopause.

***

The next day, determined to keep her training on track, Samantha contacted James with a proposal for two back-to-back fifteen-mile hikes. They would be the perfect opportunity to break in her new walking boots. Given the challenging north coast terrain, she estimated each hike would take five to six hours. They agreed on a 5 a.m. start, so they'd be home by noon.

***

The morning air was fresh, the pace good, and everything went smoothly.

Until it didn't.

At around the halfway point, Samantha's feet were on fire. She stopped to put on a blister plaster, while James reached into his backpack and offered her an energy bar. They sat munching side by side for a couple of minutes, then set off again.

An hour later, Samantha's gut started to churn. Cramps hit. Then came the dreaded sound.

She hoped James hadn't heard, but he just laughed it off. "Better out than in," he commented with a broad smile.

But it was no joke. Samantha picked up the pace until she was almost power walking, her eyes darting around for a suitable rock. She thought of Dr Pat and her pendulous poo bag. Did Samantha even have one in her backpack? Would it be any use if she did? This was code red. She instructed James to turn up the volume on his headphones to drown out any offensive acoustics, sped off the path, and managed to find a secluded spot near the cliff edge.

She made it just in time, unbuttoning her trousers and crouching down in one swift movement. Because what followed was *volcanic* diarrhoea. A veritable poonami. Only when it finally stopped did she remember that she hadn't packed any biodegradable toilet paper.

Oh shit. Literally.

Karen cackled. "You loser. James has probably already christened you Miss Poopy Pants. Better get used to it. I'm sure he'll tell everyone on the trek all about this."

"Shut up, Karen," Samantha muttered as she frantically searched through her bag.

Relief came in the form of some scented tissues. She used them with the elegance of a desperate woman in survival mode, then buried the evidence under a rock as if hiding a murder weapon. A few squirts of hand sanitizer were followed by a dab of perfume behind each ear.

Dignity, Samantha. A shred of it, anyway. You deserve that much.

James was calm and kind when she returned, his face expressing genuine concern. "Maybe we should skip tomorrow's walk?" he suggested.

"I'm fine," she insisted. "Blisters and a dodgy stomach can't stop me. I'll be there. What about you?"

Chapter 10
The Return of the Lousy Dosser

When Samantha woke up the next morning, the blisters on her feet were stinging. Her legs and shoulders ached. Her bum was … tender. But all of those gripes were to be expected. What really worried her was the dull, stabbing pain in her lower right side. Especially as it was still there when she met James at the car park.

"You okay, Princess?" he teased.

"Yeah, just sore from yesterday," she replied, forcing a smile.

But the pain increased with every step. Sweat started to trickle down her back. After another mile, nausea hit like a tidal wave. She hunched over, forcing a clenched fist into her side.

James rushed over. "Samantha, you're clearly not okay." Without hesitation, he took out his phone and called for help.

Then everything went blurry. The last thing she remembered was James catching her as she collapsed.

***

Samantha awoke in hospital, groggy and disorientated. She squinted until she could make out the figure standing at the foot or her bed. Of course, it had to be Dr Heart, her signature blend of mild concern and exasperated disapproval etched on her face.

"How are you feeling?" she said softly.

"Been better," Samantha managed.

"James told me what happened yesterday. Why didn't you come and see me? You do realize you could have died?"

"What? From a little walk in the hills? That would have been a bit dramatic, even for me, don't you think?" Samantha chuckled, then winced at the pain in her abdomen. But it was different now. More like a cut than an ache.

Before the GP could answer, Karen started bombarding Samantha with questions. "How did you get here? Did James drug you? Are your organs on eBay? Will Dr Heartless stop you going to Vietnam?"

Samantha shushed the voice in her head and demanded, "What's going on?"

"Appendicitis," Dr Heart replied, matter-of-factly. "It was very close to bursting. You were fortunate James was with you, and that you were on an accessible part of the cliff. The emergency services got you here just in time."

Samantha shuddered as she realized just how lucky she'd been. Then another thought occurred to her. "Could that have been the cause of my other symptoms?"

"Certainly."

"So … I'm not menopausal?"

"Apparently not," said Dr Heart. "Which means you owe me a lemon drizzle cake. But I won't hold you to it immediately. You should make a full recovery, but you need to rest. No baking … and no cliff hikes for the foreseeable future."

Samantha exhaled. "I guess that means you'll be rejoining the Vietnam trek?"

Dr Heart raised a quizzical eyebrow as she processed what Samantha had said. "Were you under the impression that I withdrew from the trek because of you? Whatever gave you that idea?"

Swallowing hard, Samantha whispered, "Eloise told me you were worried about a narcissist in the group. Someone who'd rub people up the wrong way. I just assumed …"

Dr Heart seemed stunned, and even a little hurt. "Believe it or not, I think I'd actually enjoy a week or two away with you. You'd certainly keep me entertained. You understand I can't reveal the identity of the actual fly in the ointment, but I'm sure you'll figure it out once you're fit enough to resume the group walks."

"So you're not banning me from going on the trek?"

"Of course not! Appendicitis is serious, but there's plenty of time for you to get back to full fitness. Just don't try to do too much too soon."

At that moment, at least half of the staff of SOS burst through the door, bearing flowers, chocolates, even homecooked meals. Samantha's face lit up, and it wasn't long before she was issuing instructions. She caught a glimpse of Dr Heart shaking her head as she left the room, but they had a big contract to win, so doctor's orders would just have to wait till later.

Once everyone had left, she messaged James: "Thanks for everything. I guess I should have listened to you after yesterday's ... incident."

He replied: "I'll swing by tomorrow during visiting hours. I've WhatsApped the rest of the group to let them know what happened this morning. Don't worry, the events of the previous day will remain our little secret 💩! Everyone's very sympathetic. Although, as ever, that woman I told you about somehow managed to bring it back to herself. Her message read like one long plug for her company. It was all 'LD Consultants this, LD Consultants that.'"

Samantha stared at her phone, then typed: "Oh my God. I know her. Her name's not Loz or Lola. It's Lorena. Otherwise known as the Lousy Dosser."

Chapter 11

The Cheerleading Squad

The following morning, Samantha felt much better physically. Emotionally was a different story.

The trek had been one of the few bright spots in her life since the loss of her mum. It had been a goal beyond work, something bigger than herself. And it had led directly to an unexpected, rewarding friendship with James.

Now, though, as she listened to Karen's latest diatribe – "Bloody Lousy Dosser! Feckin' typical of her to ruin this. Why does she even want to go on the trek? Her sole aim in life seems to be to make your life a misery!" – she felt utterly deflated. She may have bested her nemesis at the auction, but Lorena had had the last laugh. She'd be on the plane to Vietnam with the rest of the group, while Samantha would be stuck here with no one. No family. No safety net.

She opened her eyes to see James walking through the door and managed a weak smile before saying, "Thank you so much for saving my life."

"That's a bit overdramatic, darling … but you're welcome."

"Seriously, I'm eternally grateful. For calling for help, getting me off the cliff, and …" She trailed off, her eyes dropping to the floor.

James looked puzzled.

"And for your discretion."

James pinched his lips together. "I told you. That's our little secret. And I'd be quite happy never to speak of it again. *Ever*."

"Deal."

Samantha suddenly noticed a figure standing in the doorway.

James followed her gaze and beckoned the man towards them. "Introductions seem to be in order," he said, beaming. "Samantha, this is Richard, my better half. Richard, this is my crazy, funny, beautiful walking partner, Samantha."

"Lovely to meet you, Richard," said Samantha in a tone of stunned but genuine delight.

"You too," Richard replied with a soft, warm smile. "Jem has told me so much about you that I insisted on meeting you. Sounds like we've got a lot in common."

James had not given the slightest indication that he was in a relationship, but seeing them together made her heart swell. They were so at ease with each other – like Ant and Dec.

"I hope you don't mind, Sammie," said James, "but I've asked Richie to help with your recovery. I need to get you back on your feet asap. You've only been out of action a couple of days and I'm already having withdrawal symptoms."

Karen immediately pounced. "Sammie? Only me and your mother have ever called you Sammie. He's crossed a line!"

Samantha might have agreed if anyone else had tried it. But coming from James, it made her feel ... special. "Great," she said. "So, Richard, what do you do?"

"Please, *Sammie*, call me Richie," he said with a grin. "I'm not a doctor, a physio, or even a shrink. I'm a cheerleading coach."

Samantha felt her jaw drop, but no words came out.

"That means I can help with your fitness, stamina, even your gait. I hear you've been suffering from blisters." He exchanged a conspiratorial glance with James. "I can sort them out. It's what I do. Fun fact – I coached Christian Grey. Well, the actor who played him anyway. You know, in *Fifty Shades*. The Irish fella. I taught him how to walk properly, although you'd never know it from his interview with Jonathan Ross. Told him all about it, he did, but never mentioned my name. Rude."

"Oh my God," said Samantha. "I saw that show. I've been trying to copy him!"

Richie sighed, turned to James, and asked, "How's that going?"

Without missing a beat, James replied, "Not well. She looks like Bambi on ice … in boots."

Samantha giggled. She didn't usually enjoy being the butt of the joke, but she loved it with these two.

As they continued to chat, the conversation turned to hiking snacks.

"I'm a sucker for energy bars," said James. "Sammie's fond of them, too. They keep her regular. Isn't that right, Sammie?"

She groaned. "Stop! You'll make me split my sides. Literally!"

To change the subject, she started singing:

> Oh, I think that I found myself a cheerleader
> She is always right there when I need her..

James and Richie joined in, quickly adapting the lyrics:

> *He* is always right there when I need *him* …

Richie added, "You know one of the other lines in that song is 'She walks like a model,' right?"

"One step at a time," cautioned James. "I'd be happy if you could just get her walking in a straight line."

"I told you that walk of yours is ridiculous," said Karen. "They've obviously been laughing at you behind your back."

A few weeks ago, Samantha might have believed her. But something had shifted since she'd met James. She knew he'd never laugh at her. Or judge her. Or drag her down. Those were Karen's jobs. But not any more. It was time for Samantha to fight back and stand up for herself. She'd been handed a second chance. A new outlook. Even a cool war wound. And she'd recruited a couple of loyal allies.

"I'm in your hands," she said. "Now, when do we start?"

Chapter 12
Richie and Nico:
The Dynamic Duo

The doctors told Samantha that full recovery would take around six weeks. They insisted she shouldn't go into the office, but reluctantly agreed that she could work from home. So, within a few days, she was back at her desk in the home office she'd created during COVID. But there was still plenty of time for regular chats with Richie and James, either in person or on the phone.

She'd started opening up to them, even sharing stories about her mum. And she eventually provided full details of the poonami story, some of which not even James had heard before. Richie looked horrified before doubling over with laughter.

However, most of their conversations revolved around her attempts to perfect what they called the "model walk".

Whenever Samantha found herself struggling on one of the short circuits of her neighbourhood she was doing to build up her strength, she'd tell herself, "Just keep swimming, just keep swimming ..." – like Dory in *Finding Nemo*.

To which Richie would add: "Walk like a model. Own your terrain. Be the best Bambi you can be."

They spent hours coming up with new songs and chants to keep her motivated. One of the early ones went:

> Just keep swimming, just keep striving,
> With every step, just keep thriving!
> Gooooooo ... Sammie!

Initially, this was followed by the traditional "Give me an S ... Give me an A ...", but even Richie felt that was a bit over the top. Nevertheless, he continued to insist on the use of pompoms, for what he termed the "visual drama".

One favourite chant borrowed from Michael Jackson's "You Are Not Alone", which set the rhythm for many of their walks together. Richie knew Samantha needed emotional strength even more than physical stamina, so he and James would shout:

> You are not alone, we are here to cheer,
> Together we will conquer,
> You do not need to fear!

Although Richie always ensured that these training sessions were lots of fun, he was a professional who took great pride in his work. From the very start, he'd told Samantha, "Your safety comes first, but make no mistake, we're going to turn you into a trek queen." He conducted a full skills assessment, which included having her parade up and down in front of him in her hiking boots. She started with Walk #2, followed by Walk #1, and finally Walk #3. Richie watched in silence and increasing amazement ... then dropped his head into his hands.

"Oh ... my ... God. Oh my *actual* God. For the love of Jesus, can you please just show me your *normal* walk?"

Karen had been more supportive since that day in the hospital, but she could still have her moments, and this was one of them. "It's not hard, Sammie. Just put one foot in front of the other, you idiot."

"Feck off!" Samantha snapped aloud. "I know how to feckin' walk!"

Fortunately, Richie was still too busy shaking his head in disbelief to hear.

***

As Samantha's fitness increased, Richie started choreographing routines that combined longer walks with coordinated cheer moves. Before long, he had her strutting through the streets like she was on a fashion-show runway.

"Model mode, Sammie! Sass it up! Own your terrain!"

Whenever her energy started to dip, he would instruct her to shift to the "Zombie Shuffle": "Drag those feet! Arms out in front! Keep your core strong!"

Samantha would groan dramatically and laugh until she wheezed.

Every session ended with Richie yelling, "Hands in the air, cheer like you just don't care, Sammie!"

And she would. Because she didn't.

Each walk became more than exercise. It was healing. Joyful. Empowering.

The only other person who was guaranteed to make her feel that way was Nico Childs.

A mentor as much as a friend, he was a remarkably successful, self-made billionaire with a heart of gold who'd recognized her potential from the moment she'd stepped into the professional world. After guiding her through the challenges of setting up SOS, he'd celebrated each and every one of her successes as if they were his own. He was also extraordinarily patient and encouraging, even when her ideas were as ridiculous as Walk #2.

For instance, on one occasion, she told him she'd come up with a brilliant money-making scheme: selling time!

"Imagine a world where every minute is seventy-five seconds long," she explained. "There'd be so much more time to enjoy your coffee, finish that book, or simply relax."

Nico stared at her, but her pitch was bold and imaginative, and he was enjoying it, so he urged her to continue.

"We'll develop a global network of synchronized clocks that add the extra fifteen seconds to every minute. People can subscribe to our service and sync their devices to our 'Extended Time' network."

The marketing strategy would be equally audacious. "We'll target busy professionals, parents, students. Our slogan? 'More Time, More Life'. We'll create a sense of urgency – pun intended – by highlighting how precious time is and explaining how our service will give everyone more of it."

Only when he was sure she'd finished did Nico point out some of the problems with the plan. "What about the impact on global timekeeping, schedules, technology? How do you expect everyone to adjust to a whole new concept of time? And what about those who refuse to pay?"

Undeterred, Samantha replied, "We'll start with a pilot program in a small city, gather data, and refine our approach before a global rollout."

"Terrific. And once you've sold time, maybe you should try to sell patience. Lord knows, the world – and especially you, Samantha – need more of that. Don't take this the wrong way, but for someone so successful, you can be really thick sometimes."

This was typical of their conversations. Nico always knew exactly what to say to bring her back down to earth without shattering her confidence.

It was the same when she told him about the trek. He just smiled and said, "Good luck. You're going to need it."

Shortly before Easter, completely unannounced as usual, he swept into her home, squeezed her hand, and asked, "How are you feeling?" His kind, warm eyes radiated deep concern. "Your message scared the hell out of me. I thought we may have lost you." Then he took a step back and looked her up and down. "Now I can see I needn't have worried, though. This new exercise regime – what do you call it, 'cheerleader trekking'? – is obviously working wonders. You look like a different person. More relaxed."

"I feel great," she said. "But guess what?"

Nico's smile faded. "What?" he asked warily.

"The Lousy Dosser has signed up to do the Vietnam trek."

Nico rolled his eyes. "Nothing that woman does will ever surprise me." He paused for a second. "I wasn't going to mention this until you'd fully recovered, but you know that contract you've been working on? Well, she's bidding for it too. And apparently her pitch is excellent. As good as yours."

Samantha took a moment to digest the news. It was impossible to hide her disappointment. "Really? As good as mine?" she asked, her throat tightening.

Nico rested a reassuring hand on her arm. "Listen to me, Samantha. You're brilliant. You've built an amazing team. It'll be fine." He hugged her tightly. "Now, get some rest. I'll see you again soon." He made his way to the front door and closed it behind him.

For the first time in weeks, Samantha felt truly alone.

Karen whispered darkly, "Prepare for war. The Lousy Dosser is coming for you again!"

Chapter 13

A New Lease of Life

Samantha had always been an avid collector of random trivia. One morning, as she sipped her turmeric latte, a strange but inspiring fact popped into her head: Pope Francis used to be a nightclub bouncer.

She chuckled to herself. *Well, if he can go from tossing drunk lads out of clubs to running the Vatican, surely I can go from spreadsheets to something more meaningful. I mean, who says I can't be the next Lhakpa Sherpa and summit Everest ten times?*

Karen couldn't let that one go. "Yeah, right. You get altitude sickness on a step ladder."

Since her brush with death – "Drama queen!" Richie's voice echoed through her head – and the growing threat from the Lousy Dosser, Samantha had been more determined than ever to overhaul every aspect of her life – physical, emotional, and spiritual.

As her mum used to say, "You only get one life, Sammie. So you should enjoy yourself. Spend your money. Make memories. You can't take it with you. And even if you could, there's no Mulberry in the afterlife."

Moreover, despite the occasional lapse back into negativity, for the most part, Karen had transformed herself into an equally effective motivational speaker. "Don't talk, act! Don't say, do! Don't promise, prove!" She would even start belting out "Let it go! Let it go!" from *Frozen* whenever Samantha started mulling over past regrets.

Part of this personal reinvention was a grocery list that now read like a page from Gwyneth Paltrow's blog leafy greens, fermented foods, chia seeds – but Samantha knew that most of the credit for her newfound energy had to go to James and Richie. Karen called her their "pet project", and while she hated the term, she had to admit that they had trained her well. Without them, she probably would have been languishing in bed, feeling sorry for herself, rather than striding through the streets with ever more confidence and self-belief.

Their five-year relationship was still so full of love, humour, passion, and honest openness. Seeing them together conjured up wistful memories of her own relationship history: Nathan, her sweet high-school love; Fin, the dependable college partner; and, of course, Kev, who'd remained close to her mum even after their split, dropping by every Wednesday for beef-and-beetroot sandwiches and Tayto crisps. He hated the crisps, but was always too polite to say so.

There'd been no shortage of offers to take Kev's place, but she'd chosen to remain single ever since. Clumsy kisses, bad breath, roaming hands – she could do without the dating merry-go-round, thank you very much.

Karen's probing grew louder with each passing year: "You'll make a great cat mum, but are you sure that's the only relationship you want?"

Samantha didn't have an answer. But she did really like cats.

Chapter 14

Working 7 to 9, What a Way to Make a Living

Nico's intel proved to be spot on.

Lorena Dean, the Lousy Dosser, had indeed struck again. Like a smug, cackling hyena, she'd swooped in and snatched a high-profile contract from right from under Samantha's nose.

This wasn't just business. This was personal.

Samantha's stomach churned as she went through the details of the bidding process. What she was feeling was more than professional disappointment. Something was off. How had Lorena managed to undercut her? How had her pitch mirrored Samantha's so closely?

Naturally, Karen had a number of suggestions: "She's planted a mole in your office. Or bugged your laptop. Or implanted a microchip in your brain. I told you not to use free Wi-Fi in coffee shops. This is industrial espionage!"

As the seeds of doubt took root and started to sprout, everything in the office suddenly seemed suspicious. Overly formal emails. Side glances that lingered too long. Casual conversations laced with subtext. What had once been trusted colleagues were now suspects.

She found herself working all hours of the day, seven days a week, in an effort to claw back control. Had she taken her eye off the ball? Was this cosmic punishment for starting to enjoy life again? She'd built the business from nothing, weathered previous storms, heartbreak, and betrayals, but this this felt like someone had stolen a piece of her soul.

Her sleep suffered. Her walking routine crumbled. Her energy levels plummeted.

The idea that someone in her circle might be working against her made her feel physically sick. But who could it be?

"Well, let's look at the most likely candidates," chirped Karen. "That bright as a button intern? Nobody's *that* keen. Or Hayden from HR? She's been giving you the stink eye for weeks."

"Stop it!" shouted Samantha into the darkness of her bedroom. Then again, now she thought about it, Hayden had been unusually chatty recently.

She pounded her head with her palm. Her paranoia was becoming relentless. Every time she thought about Lorena's smug, lip-glossed face, the knot in her chest twisted tighter.

The Lousy Dosser was chipping away at her business, her self-confidence, her peace of mind.

Enough was enough. Something had to be done.

***

Samantha's first tactic was covert surveillance. She stood with her ear pressed against her office door, at one point even trying that old trick of using a glass as an amplifier, but it made no difference – she still heard nothing. Then she casually left the door open, waited till no one was looking, and crouched under her desk. She got cramp after five minutes. Finally, she locked herself in one of the toilet cubicles, stood on the seat, and waited for the traitors to enter and discuss their crime. They never did.

Next, she created a fake proposal and told her team it was strictly confidential. Not a single leak.

***

A few days later, two senior members the team, Alex and Cris, entered her office to find her slumped at her desk, her hands balled into fists.

"Are you okay?" Alex asked tentatively.

"Do I look okay, Alex?" she barked.

Alex stood frozen, his mouth slightly open. Cris furrowed her brows.

"Sorry," said Samantha. "But losing that contract to LD has really got to me. The bidding process was supposed to be confidential, yet their proposal was almost identical to ours. Just a bit cheaper."

"But how? We're always so careful to keep everything under wraps," said Alex.

"You tell me," said Samantha, her voice shaking.

Alex exchanged a glance with Cris. "Do you think there's a mole in the office?"

Samantha sighed, running a hand through her tangled hair. "God knows, I don't *want* to think that. But what else could it be?"

Cris stepped forward, firm but kind. "Sam, you know you can trust us. We'll help you figure this out. If we need to do some … investigating, then let's do it."

Alex nodded. As the tech lead, he knew the firm's systems inside out. "We can start by reviewing who had full access to the pitch. Don't worry. I'm onto it."

Samantha felt a flicker of hope. "Thanks, guys. I really appreciate it. This has to end."

"We'll get through this together," promised Cris.

Alex added softly, "Absolutely. Remember, you're not alone."

Samantha took a deep breath and steeled herself. "All right. Let's do this. Time to take back control."

***

That evening, she met James and Richie for dinner. Colleagues were all well and good, but right now she needed some friends.

Inevitably, though, the conversation soon turned to the search for the mole.

"I'm sure your team will leave no stone unturned," said Richie. "But it wouldn't hurt to do a little digging of your own." His eyes drifted towards James, who gave a slight nod. "A few years ago," Richie continued, "we were in need of the services of a private detective." Samantha's eyes widened. "I won't bore you with the details, but suffice to say he was excellent. Would you like his contact details?"

Samantha hesitated, but relented when Richie held up his phone, sighing, "Okay, send them over." Her own phone pinged a couple of seconds later.

Back at home, reasoning she couldn't be too careful, she contacted the detective using her Katie Green account.

In her imagination, he was a Jack Reacher type. Ruggedly handsome, ex-military, a brooding loner. Dangerous but ethical with a dark past and an enigmatic smile. He'd swoop in and solve the case in twenty-four hours or less.

His name was Kevin Reece Jones. Richie had described him as calm, steady, dependable, a good problem-solver.

"Maybe it's something about the name?" muttered Samantha with a smile. Her ex could have been described in exactly the same way.

In her message to Kevin, she suggested meeting at a quiet café just outside of town. Tomorrow, if that would work for him.

He replied with a 👍 emoji and a PDF attachment containing a breakdown of his fees.

Chapter 15

How to Catch a Rat

The bell above the café door jingled.

Samantha looked up. Then froze. Her heart slammed hard against her chest.

"Kev?" she breathed.

Still tall. Still broad-shouldered. Still *those* eyes, although time had written itself into the creases at their corners. He looked like someone who'd lived fully and loved deeply.

"Wow," Karen swooned. "He's aged. But like a fine whiskey. Drink him in, Sammie."

"Sam?" Kev's startled face instantly softened into a combination of joy and bemusement. "Wow. What are you doing here?"

She didn't know whether to laugh, cry, or fling herself into his arms.

Especially when he said, "I heard about your mum. I'm so sorry. She was a great lady."

They fell into silence, lost in memories of beef-and-beetroot sandwiches and cheese-and-onion Taytos.

After what seemed like hours, he finally stammered, "Of course, I think about you, too."

Same old Kev, thought Samantha. He always had a tendency to over-share when he was nervous.

"I wish I could chat," he said, suddenly businesslike, "but I'm meeting someone here. Maybe we could grab a drink later? Or not. Just a thought."

"Meeting someone?" echoed Samantha. "Kev ... are you Kevin Reece Jones?"

"Yes. In my line of work it pays to use a pseudonym," he said, clearly reciting a line he'd delivered a thousand times before. "But ..."

"I'm Katie Green," said Samantha, stretching out a clammy, trembling hand. "Pleased to meet you, Kevin."

Instinctively, Kev seized her hand, shook it briskly, then quickly released it. "Sam, what the fuck is going on?" he asked, eyes wide.

Samantha couldn't find the words. All she could think was: *After all this time, here he is. My Kev. My hero. Standing in front of me. Ready to spring into action and fix everything.*

***

They talked for hours. Kev explained that he'd gone into the private detective business a couple of years after they'd split up, while Samantha filled him in on SOS. That led naturally to the reason why she'd contacted him. She handed over a ring binder containing all the evidence she'd collected so far. He listened carefully, taking copious notes.

Finally, he said, "Well, that's more than enough to be getting on with. Now, how about that drink? Or a bite to eat?"

Samantha hesitated. She was terrified. Of reopening doors that had been locked for years. Of allowing herself to feel vulnerable. Of hurting him. "Best not," she said. "We've got a rat to catch. Maybe once it's safely in the trap?"

"No problem," said Kev, although his eyes betrayed his disappointment. "I'll get cracking and give you an update in a few days' time. How about Friday? Same time, same place?"

Samantha nodded. "Perfect."

They shook hands awkwardly and went their separate ways … again.

***

In the office the next morning, Samantha watched everyone with a keen detective's eye. Emotionally detached but alert, she studied their movements, their body language, and their choice of words. Someone, somewhere, had betrayed her, and she was determined to find out who.

This wasn't just any office. It was *her* office. *Her* business. The one she had poured blood, sweat, and tears into. The one that had cost her countless sleepless nights, holidays, and relationships, including the one with Kev.

And yet, even though they both knew it had caused the rift between them, he'd selflessly agreed to save SOS. Because he knew how much it meant to her.

Karen wasn't so sure. "Admit it, Sammie, you've taken your eye off the ball. Having fun with James and Richie. Focusing all your attention on the trek. Do you really have any idea what your team have been doing for the last six months. Do you even know all of their names?"

Some of the barbs stung, not least because Samantha knew they were true.

***

On Friday, they found a secluded corner of the café and Kev fired up his laptop. Angling the screen so they both could see it, he said, "Ready?"

Samantha nodded.

He'd combed through all the data she'd provided – emails, internal comms, security footage, server access logs, HR reports – and emerged with three prime suspects:

> 1. Mary: The well-meaning account manager who'd suggested Samantha might be menopausal. "Something seems a bit off," said Kev. "Always first in, last out. She's working more hours than the rest of the team, so maybe some of them are on behalf of someone else."

2. Jax: The newbie. Video footage showed him lingering outside Samantha's office on more than one occasion and furiously texting afterwards. He'd been hired specifically to work on the pitch for the contract that they'd lost to LD.

3. Aine: One of SOS's longest-serving employees, a single mum of three, and someone Samantha had always trusted implicitly. Lately, though, she seemed a bit distracted. "There's a new boyfriend on the scene," Kev noted. "I've not looked into him yet, but I will."

***

On Monday morning, after a weekend of trying to figure out the best course of action, Samantha called an impromptu meeting of her leadership team. It was a risky move, but she needed allies, so she felt she had to come clean with them.

"Scumbag!" shouted Liam, the excitable sales director, when Samantha explained that they'd almost certainly lost the contract because of an internal security breach. "How could someone do that to us?"

"Got me," replied Samantha. "But the wheels are already in motion to track them down. Alex, how are you getting on?"

"Nothing yet," said Alex. "But it's early days. Hang in there. We'll find them."

That was the signal for the rest of the team to rally around. It was like a locker room after a crushing defeat: shellshocked, angry, protective, but most of all united.

This was her team. The one she'd recruited. She looked at each of their faces in turn and saw nothing but undivided loyalty.

And yet …

***

At their next meeting, Kev flipped open the laptop and brought up the dossiers on each of the prime suspects in turn.

- Mary's long hours? Entirely legitimate. She was a workaholic, not a weasel.
- Jax's strange behaviour? First-week nerves and an overly concerned partner who texted him supportive messages on the hour, every hour.
- Aine? The boyfriend wasn't a corporate spy but a clingy romantic who insisted on hours of late-night FaceTime. Aine wasn't a traitor; she was exhausted.

Then Kev opened a new file and tapped the screen. "*This* is your rat."

In capital letters at the top of the screen was a single word: "ALEX".

"Nooooo!" cried Samantha.

Kev scrolled through the evidence. It had been buried, encrypted, disguised, but he'd managed to decode it, and it was damning.

Alex had been feeding sensitive information to the Lousy Dosser for regular kickbacks and the promise of a senior position at LD once SOS had been driven into the dust. But the biggest kicker was that he was clearly in love with her. Reading through their emails, it was obvious to Samantha that Lorena didn't feel the same way, but she'd been stringing him along for months.

When Samantha confronted him, her voice was shaking with fury. "Why did you do this, Alex? There's no other word for it. You betrayed us."

He didn't answer.

She raised a finger, full *Apprentice* style. "You're fired. Now, get out of my office. I never want to see you again."

A sneer started to spread across Alex's lips. "Ahh, Sam, I'm afraid you don't always get what you want. You will be seeing me again. Quite soon. At an employment tribunal. This is unfair dismissal."

Before the meeting, Samantha had asked Hayden to wait outside, as a witness in case Alex started making unfounded accusations. Now, without even bothering to knock, the HR officer burst through the door. "No problem, Alex," she said. "We would welcome a tribunal. A licensed private investigator has submitted a detailed report on your activities. Here's a copy." She coolly handed it over. "I think you'll need a good lawyer."

Alex paled and left without another word.

Samantha rose from behind her desk and threw her arms around Hayden. "Thank you. You were amazing!"

Hayden grinned. "So were you. That finger point? I've fired a few people in my time but I've never had the nerve to do it."

"He deserved it. This year has been hell."

"Agreed. He's a cocky little shit. But don't let him get under your skin. Everyone else here adores you. Including me."

Samantha smiled, genuinely touched, then wondered how she could have been so wrong about Hayden.

***

With Kev's help, Samantha set up new security protocols, ensured the whole team changed their passwords, and recruited a temporary IT expert to plug the gap left by Alex's departure.

With the rat caught, she could finally breathe again. Her body, mind, and business had all been through the wringer, but now she could focus on what was really important.

Healing.

Rebuilding.

And walking.

She knew the pain of losing her mum would never go away. But the trek might help. She vowed to complete it in her mother's honour.

The ache for Kev was just as persistent, but different. She found herself thinking of him most nights. The old memories whispered, "What if …?" Sometimes, her finger hovered over his phone number, ready to call, ready to ask, "How about that drink?" But then fear would always take over. Well, fear … and Karen.

"Leave the past in the past," she would snarl. "Don't be a feckin' idiot, Sammie."

Maybe she was right, but Samantha made a promise to herself. After the trek, she would make the call. Just coffee. No pressure. No drama. Just verification.

She had to know if what she was feeling was real or a lethal cocktail of hope and nostalgia.

She took a deep breath and smiled.

The worst was behind her. The trek lay ahead.

And she was ready.

One step at a time.

Chapter 16

The Real Adventure Begins

Samantha loved Hanoi. Or at least, she *wanted* to love it.

Vietnam's capital certainly lived up to its reputation. It was steeped in history, culture, and charm. But "bustling" wasn't the half of it. The place was a complete sensory overload. Simply crossing the street reminded her of that old arcade game, Frogger. Except you had only one life. Forget five lanes, try thirty. Scooters, bicycles, motorbikes, flower carts, chickens, fruit stalls, a rogue piglet or two. It was chaos incarnate.

The colours were vibrant, the beeping horns relentless, the brakes screeching, the locals yelling, laughing, chanting, and singing. It was as if the entire city was in the midst of a perpetual festival.

And as for smells! Sweet Mary, Mother of God. Exhaust fumes stuck to Samantha's clothes like a clingy ex. Waves of mouthwatering aromas drifted from the food trucks, followed by sharp hits of incense wafting from temples. The last of these made her shudder, as they instantly transported her back to her mother's funeral – the last time she'd set foot inside a church. It was the one memory of her mum she didn't want. But then she'd be assaulted by some new sensation that dragged her back to the here and now. The place was just so … *alive*!

This was supposed to be the calm before the storm. A few days to relax and acclimatize before heading off to Sapa – a mountainous gem in the north of the country – where the group would trek through rice terraces, breathtaking peaks, and villages perched precariously on the hillsides. However, relaxation was in short supply, and not only during the daytime. Because on the first night Samantha learned she was sharing a room with the Lousy Dosser … and would be for the rest of the trip.

She begged Eloise for a different roommate, but the only other women in the group were Julie and Tricia (best friends who refused to be separated), Eloise herself, and Emily (aka Dr Heartless), who had finally caved and agreed to rejoin the trek after months of lobbying from her sister-in-law. Emily drew the line at sharing a room with either Samantha or Lorena, though, saying it would be "unethical" as they were both patients of hers.

Inevitably, James found the whole situation hilarious. "Sammie," he chuckled, "you know I'd bunk up with you in a heartbeat if our gracious hosts allowed it. But they're convinced that no man would be able to resist you, so they've got to keep us apart." He winked. "You never know, though. Sharing with Lorena might be good for you."

Samantha groaned. "Good for me? What, like a colonoscopy?"

Each evening, she would return to the guest house to find that Lorena had used all the hot water or dumped her sweaty boots in the middle of the room. At which point Karen would burst into a chorus of "Let it go! Let it go!"

And Samantha did ... just. But it was a struggle.

Strangely, the record changed the moment they arrived in Sapa, as Karen reverted back to motivational-speaker mode: "Don't talk, act! Don't say, do! Don't promise, prove!"

Samantha found herself chanting along under her breath. She hated to admit it, but Karen was right. Something had to be done. The tension between herself and Lorena was suffocating, and they hadn't even walked a single kilometre yet.

***

At dawn, mist hung over the ethereal rice terraces like a veil. Samantha gazed in awe as she laced up her boots, then took a long, steadying breath. Part of her hoped that Lorena had come down with a dose of Delhi – or rather Hanoi – belly during the night, but no such luck. There she was, fawning over James and asking him to adjust the straps on her backpack. He glanced over at Samantha and rolled his eyes.

Nevertheless, as they set off, he whispered, "Just talk to her. Get it out. Richie thinks it'll be therapeutic."

"Or she'll grab my walking poles and ram them in my back," Samantha muttered.

There was other advice, too. In one ear, her mother: "You can do this, Sammie. One step at a time." In the other, Karen: "This is war. Don't let your guard down for a second."

Finally, they all quietened down, which gave her an opportunity to reflect on the previous year. It had been one of grief, self-doubt, illness, healing, betrayal, redemption, new friends, and one old flame. So much had happened, but through it all she'd been spurred on by this – a trek through the stunning, hushed, sacred scenery of Vietnam. She couldn't let Lorena ruin that for her.

Just after lunch, with the emerald-green mountains spreading like a baize quilt behind them and the sun peeking through clouds, she made her way to the back of the line.

"Lorena," she said, her breath catching, "can I have a word?"

Lorena just kept looking straight ahead, eyes slightly narrowed, as if Samantha didn't exist.

Karen whispered, "Well, you tried, but she's obviously not interested, so feck her."

Samantha needed to know, though. "Why did you do it? Why did you sabotage me?"

Still no response, but now she could see that Lorena was really struggling – gasping for breath, wincing with every step. Their pace had slowed to little more than a crawl.

Good! Serves you right, thought Samantha. *I hope your blisters are the size of your ego.*

They were starting to fall behind the rest of the group, and there were so many twists and turns on the narrow track that the others would momentarily disappear from view before re-emerging further up the hill. Then, suddenly, there was no sign of them.

Samantha turned to Lorena. "Brilliant. We must have taken a wrong turn. Looks like it's just the two of us. Lost in Vietnam. Together."

Chapter 17

Peace Breaks Out

They both scanned the landscape: endless rice fields, winding paths, dramatic mountaintops, and lush valleys. But no charity trekking group.

Samantha checked her phone for the fifth time and felt her frustration bubbling. "Still no feckin' signal. Typical. And of all the people I could have been stranded with, why did it have to be you?"

Lorena huffed and crossed her arms, mirroring Samantha's irritation. "Oh, please. I'm hardly thrilled about this, either. But standing around bitching about it isn't going to summon a GPS from the sky, is it?"

"Jaysus, it speaks!" screamed Karen. "Just listen to her. Acting all practical."

Samantha knew that the Lousy Dosser was right, though. "Don't talk, act," she muttered under her breath.

They tried – and failed – to retrace their steps as the sun dipped ever lower in the sky, casting golden shadows over the rice terraces. With the light fading fast, Lorena's trademark smugness started to mutate into breathless panic. And she'd taken to hobbling along on the edges of her boots in a vain attempt to relieve the pain of the blisters.

Eventually, Samantha could take no more of it. As dusk turned to night, she grabbed Lorena's arm and said, "Stop! This is pointless. We're never going to find them now. We'll figure it out in the morning."

Lorena, seemingly relieved that the decision had been made for her, slumped down against the trunk of a nearby tree.

"Your feet okay?" asked Samantha.

Lorena winced as she hauled off her boots. "These socks have been cutting into me like razor wire. I hardly dare look."

Without a word, Samantha opened her backpack, pulled out some foot powder, fresh socks, and blister plasters, then placed them in front of Lorena like peace offerings.

Then she excused herself for a much-needed pee, muttering her mother's old adage: "It's nice to be nice."

When she returned, she lay on the ground, rested her head on her backpack, and stared into the night sky.

The silence stretched out like elastic between them until Lorena finally snapped it.

"You know, I never really wanted to start my own consultancy." Her voice was soft, hesitant. "I only did it because I felt like I had to prove myself. You were always this

… force of nature. Highly respected. Confident. I wanted that. I wanted to *be* that."

"Liar, liar, pants on fire," sang Karen.

Samantha folded her arms. "And the way to achieve that was to sabotage me?"

"I didn't sabotage you," Lorena spluttered, as if the words had just been Heimliched out of her lungs. "I didn't steal the contract. I just submitted my pitch and won it, fair and square."

Samantha's jaw tightened. "But the structure, the wording, the budget. They were all virtually identical to my proposal."

Lorena shrugged. "I worked for you for years, remember. Do you think I didn't learn anything?"

"But you kept learning from me even after you left SOS, didn't you?" It was time to play her trump card. "I know all about your little mole. Alex!"

"Let's see her weasel her way out of that one," said Karen.

"Mole?" said Lorena, genuinely perplexed. "Alex was in financial trouble, so I helped him out by sending a few little tech jobs his way. While he was working on them, he suggested some new approaches and frameworks. They were good ideas, so we implemented them. He took full credit for them. I had no idea they'd come from you. Honestly, if I'd known, I never would have used them."

Samantha exhaled as she reflected on what she'd just heard. It seemed plausible. But if it were true, if Lorena had borne her no ill-will, why had she tried to outbid her at the auction, and then signed up for the trek anyway? "Okay, given everything you've said, why are you here? You must have known it would be awkward between us."

Lorena paused. "I didn't come because of you," she said, her voice barely more than a whisper. "I came because of my dad. He's been diagnosed with Parkinson's. Jersey Cheshire is helping him and dozens like him. That's why I bid so much at the auction. I wanted to give a bit back."

"I'm so sorry to hear that," Samantha said gently. "How's your mum coping?"

Lorena looked up, startled by the unexpected kindness. "Okay, I guess. Struggling, but trying to stay strong."

At that moment, James's unmistakable voice echoed through the darkness. "Sammie? Lorena?"

Both women froze for a second before jumping to their feet. Then they both started waving their torches like madwomen and shouting at the tops of their voices.

Within minutes, Eloise, James, and Emily materialized from the shadows, equal parts relieved and amused.

Eloise raised an eyebrow. "I half expected to find one of you buried under the rice paddies and the other standing by with a shovel. But this all seems remarkably civilized."

"We've called a ceasefire," said Samantha.

James slapped Samantha on the back and said, "See? Miracles do happen."

The force of the slap, coupled with the fatigue in her legs after a hard day's trekking, sent Samantha spinning to the ground. She emerged moments later with two streaks of mud under each eye.

"You badass," said Karen. "Bambi's turned into Rambo."

Samantha liked the sound of that. It suited her. She felt stronger. Fitter.

She could handle this. All of it.

Chapter 18

Second Chances

After they arrived at the guest house, Samantha spent what remained of the evening replaying Lorena's words in her mind, turning them over like smooth stones. Could she forgive her? Could she move on from all the bitterness, betrayal, and bruised pride? The weight of grief, exhaustion, and rage had clung to her like a second skin for years. Tonight, she finally felt like she might be able to shed it.

She stared at the ceiling of their shared room, listening to the steady rhythm of Lorena's breathing from across the room. "I believe you," she said softly into the darkness.

A pause. The sound of rustling sheets. Then a fragile voice: "You do?"

Samantha swallowed the lump that had formed in her throat. "Yeah. I do. I'm sorry for doubting you."

A breath of relief floated across the room. Followed by a barely audible "Thank you."

The dam had been breached.

They talked for hours. About work. About the past. About regrets and colossal mistakes. Emotions ran high. There were gales of laughter and floods of tears.

At one point, Lorena asked, "Do you still think about your mum?"

The question hit Samantha like a sucker punch. "Every second of every day."

Lorena nodded. "I can't imagine how …" Her voice trailed off into silence.

"The thing about devastating loss," said Samantha carefully, "is that life keeps going. That leaves you with a choice to make: you either turn with the world or you turn your back on it."

There was a long, heavily weighted pause. "And which did you choose?" Lorena asked.

Samantha felt her lips form the ghost of a smile. "I'm an orphan who's learning how to turn with the world. And trying like hell to make my parents proud."

Lorena wiped a hand across her eyes. "I'm sorry, Samantha. I never meant to hurt you. I was stupid. I never should have left."

Samantha turned her head to meet Lorena's gaze in the moonlight. For the first time in years, she didn't see a rival. She didn't see the Lousy Dosser. She saw a woman she used to trust. A woman who had once felt like family.

She said nothing. She didn't need to.

***

The next day was gruelling. After minimal sleep, Samantha and Lorena were mentally and emotionally drained. The steep climbs, slick mud trails, and relentless heat tested every ounce of their endurance.

And yet, Samantha felt lighter, liberated, free to be herself. She and James spent their breaks recording ridiculous TikTok videos of cheer chants and dance routines for Richie. The rest of the group loved it. Even Lorena cracked a smile when she wasn't attending to her blistered feet.

Then, somewhere along a ridgeline above the rice paddies – sweaty, footsore, and slightly sunburned – Samantha thought back to when Lorena had worked for her. Remembered how sharp she'd been. How full of promise. Yes, she'd been impatient, occasionally devious, painfully naive, and more than a little selfish. But she'd also been committed, creative, and passionate.

She suddenly realized what she had to do. After slowing her pace to let the others past, she fell into step with Lorena and said quietly, "I want you to come back."

Lorena was confused. "Come back? To where?"

"SOS. You'll have to start at the bottom, of course. No special treatment. No fast-tracking."

Lorena didn't need long to consider the offer. "That's fair," she said, simply. "I'd love to come back. Thank you for giving me a second chance."

"Brilliant move, Rambo," said Karen. "Keep your friends close and your enemies closer."

Samantha smiled. Time would tell if it was brilliant or not. But she felt pretty sure that Lorena was no longer an enemy.

Chapter 19
Campfire Banter

It was a trek tradition that the group would gather around the campfire each evening with a few local beers to share stories on a particular theme. Then, around 10 p.m., Eloise would give a short speech and hand out two small stuffed toys.

The first was a little plush pig – the Pig of Perfection – which was awarded for acts of exceptional courage, selflessness, or kindness. It was a light-hearted honour but increasingly coveted as the week wore on. Inevitably, James had won it on day one for tracking down Samantha and Lorena. (And, Samantha suspected, just for being himself. For God's sake, could the guy be any more perfect?)

The second was the Sheep of Shame – a goofy little creature that was the prize for the most embarrassing moment of the day. Tricia's now legendary bladder meant she was often in the running.

Tonight, the air was still, the stars bright, and the fire was casting a warm glow across their tired, dirt-smudged faces.

Samantha sat cross-legged, absently poking at the glowing embers with a stick.

Dr Emily had suggested that they should all share what had brought them to Vietnam. Thus far, roughly half of the stories had been moving, the other half hilarious.

"Lorena, you're up," said Eloise.

Lorena took a deep breath, looked around the expectant faces, then spoke for ten minutes about her father and his Parkinson's diagnosis. She said she was walking for him because one day soon, he wouldn't be able to walk at all. Her voice cracked as she described the hospital visits and her sense of helplessness as she witnessed his steady decline.

Samantha already knew much of the story from the night they'd got lost on the mountainside, but it seemed even more powerful now. Which left her feeling even more guilty for assuming that Lorena had joined the trek merely to spite her.

Dr Emily simply nodded, ever the cool, reserved GP. "Thank you, Lorena. Okay, who's left? Samantha? How about you?"

Samantha laughed awkwardly. "Well, I'm here because I was determined to outbid Lorena at an auction. That's it. Sorry – I know it's a bit boring compared to everyone else."

There were a few chuckles from the group, but James's expression was unusually serious. "Come on, Bambi," he said, gently nudging her shoulder. "Tell the real story. We've got plenty of time."

Karen started shouting, "Don't do it. They'll only judge you."

"Let them," muttered Samantha. She didn't want to hide any more.

She talked about her mum. About the shock of losing her while on holiday. About the silence that had filled her home in the aftermath. About the deep ache that was still there in the pit of her stomach.

Then she talked about her dad. About his final generous gift, which had enabled her to start her own business. About how she was both immensely proud of that business and burdened by the fear of letting him down if it failed.

She concluded with: "I guess I came on this trek because I needed to find something outside of work. Something other than grief. Something just for me. Something that might help me feel more like myself again."

Silence followed. Not tense. Just still.

"Well done, Sammie," whispered Karen.

James reached over to give her a comforting pat on the back. "Proud of you, Bambi."

Then Lorena murmured, "I'm sorry for your loss."

Similar sentiments echoed around the campfire until everyone was lost in their own thoughts.

After a respectful minute or two, Dr Emily clapped her hands together and announced, "Right, that just leaves me. Time for my story." She paused dramatically. "I came on this trek because I heard that one of the previous doctors did a dump in full view of half of Iceland, then proudly carried the poo all the way down a mountain. Well, I just had to try to top that."

As the rest of the group howled with laughter, Samantha caught her GP's eye and mouthed, "Thank you."

Emily replied with a silent, "You're welcome."

Once the laughter had subsided, Eloise rose to her feet, cleared her throat with theatrical flair, and announced, "Well, the votes have been counted, and for the first time in history, we have a double award-winner. The Pig of Perfection and the Sheep of Shame both go to … Samantha!"

Cheers erupted. James whooped. Tricia clapped, possibly relieved that she wouldn't have to find space in her backpack for yet another sheep.

Eloise grinned. "By way of explanation, you deserve the pig because it took a lot of courage to tell that story. As for the sheep … well, we now know that you're only here because you couldn't bear to lose to Lorena at the auction. You should be ashamed of yourself!"

More laughter rippled through the group as Samantha stood, bowed deeply, and accepted the two plush toys with elaborate reverence.

They were camping under the stars tonight, and it wasn't long before they were all zipping up their sleeping bags and shouting "Good night" to each other, like a scene from *The Waltons*.

Once the voices had died down, Samantha looked up at the moon and felt a swirl of emotions: raw vulnerability, relief, pride. And something she hadn't experienced in a very long time: a sense of belonging.

After what seemed like years, she was no longer alone.

Chapter 20

The Summit and the Call

The next morning, Samantha's her heart was full to bursting as she tied the Pig of Perfection and the Sheep of Shame to her backpack. She almost skipped along the path as they set off, but before long her legs and her lungs were burning. It was the final day of the trek, and the air was much thinner at this altitude. Every step felt like dragging herself through wet concrete.

James looked over his shoulder and saw that she was struggling. "Come on, Bambi," he called. "We're nearly there."

"I can't," Samantha gasped, collapsing onto a rock, her face flushed crimson. "I'm done. I'm fecked."

"Typical," scoffed Karen. "You never finish anything."

Samantha froze. Then she snapped. "No." Her voice was low but firm. "You're wrong. I *can* do this. I *will* do this. And while we're at it, I'm done listening to you."

She hauled herself to her feet, legs shaking, but determination coursing through her veins like adrenaline. She took a step. Then another. And another.

James stopped and turned to face her. "Oh my God. You look like Bambi … if Bambi had shit himself."

Samantha laughed through gritted teeth. "I don't care. Whatever it takes, I'm doing it." In her head, Richie's cheer chants played on a loop: "Just keep swimming, just keep striving …"

Then, without knowing or understanding or caring how she'd done it, she reached the peak. The sun was still rising behind her, casting long shadows across the valley below. Her breath caught in her throat. Her eyes welled with tears. "We made it, Mum," she shouted at the top of her voice. Then she whispered, "I hope I made you proud."

"Well, this is awkward," said Karen. "If you keep crying, people will think you're broken."

Maybe I am, thought Samantha. *But that's okay.*

Behind her, James muttered, "If you make me cry, I'll throw you off this bloody mountain." Then he placed a hand on her shoulder, squeezing gently. "Sammie, your mum would be *so* proud. And I'm proud of you, too, you muppet. You have no idea how completely amazing you are."

She pulled him into a tight hug and whispered, "I couldn't have done it without my early riser … and his cheerleader boyfriend." She paused for dramatic effect. "Oh, and by the way, I'm Katie Green."

James's jaw almost hit the floor. "You little witch. I've spent the last six months wondering what happened to her!"

Moments later, Eloise arrived at the summit, breathless but beaming. "Well, babes ... we did it. Well done all of you." Then she promptly lost her footing and fell into an undignified heap, breaking the emotional tension with a loud thud.

***

Spirits were high that evening at the celebration dinner. Wine flowed freely, and stories were shared with a mixture of pride and disbelief.

Samantha was several glasses in when she felt the buzz of bold decision-making like an electric current up her spine.

She leaned over to James and told him she planned to call Kev.

"Oooooh, in the mood for a bit of drunk dialling, are we?"

Samantha waved him off and knocked over the soy sauce. "It won't be drunk dialling. It'll be the result of sober reflection on my life's journey."

"Wait," said Tricia, who'd been not so subtly eavesdropping. "Is this *the* Kev? The one who got away?"

Samantha slurred, "He didn't away. *I* left *him*. And he let me go. It was all very adult and emotionally mature and ..."

"You do realize you're wearing a napkin as a cape?" James interrupted, fanning himself with a menu.

Samantha looked down, then over each shoulder. Sure enough, the napkin had somehow slipped around her neck and was now dangling down her back. With as much dignity as she could muster, she grabbed it and dropped it to the floor. "Right. I be calling now. Everyone shut up."

She brought up Kev's number and pressed CALL.

One ring. Two.

Oh God. What if this is a mistake? What if he doesn't answer? What if ... ?

"Sam?"

Her heart skipped a beat.

"Kev," she breathed.

He sounded surprised. And, unless the wine was playing tricks, pleased.

"I wasn't expecting to hear from you till next week," he said. "This is so weird, though. I almost called you yesterday."

"You did?"

Tricia slapped a hand over James's mouth to muffle the squeal that was about to escape.

Kev chuckled. "Yeah. I saw an old email from you. Had a bit of a ... nostalgic moment."

"That's not nostalgia," said Samantha, earnestly. "That's fate."

Kev paused. "Have you been drinking, Sam?"

"Yes! Lots. But that's not why I'm phoning. I'm phoning because I miss you."

There it was. She'd said it. There was no backing out now.

Another pause. Longer this time. Then: "I miss you too, Sam."

James brushed away Tricia's hand and started chanting, "It's happening, it's really happening."

"I want to hear everything," said Kev. "Where are you? What are you doing?"

"I'm in Vietnam. I've climbed actual mountains. My feet are killing me. There's no oxygen. But it's been … life-changing."

Kev laughed. That warm, familiar sound that used to melt her heart. Still melted her heart. "Sounds like quite the adventure."

"Oh, you have no idea," she said.

They talked about the trek, his work, their lives. It wasn't awkward. It was … effortless.

The rest of the group, with the exception of James and Tricia, gradually resumed their own conversations once they realized that the phone call was likely to take some time.

Finally, Kev said, "Listen, Sam, I'd love to catch up properly once you're back."

Karen shouted, "Retreat! This is how you get hurt!"

Samantha rolled her eyes. "I'd like that too, Kev."

As she hung up, Tricia and James whooped, which triggered a spontaneous round of applause from the rest of the group. Even Dr Emily was clapping. As was Lorena.

James wiped away a fake tear. "Our girl is back in the game!" He raised his glass high. "To Sammie. And Kev. He won't know what's hit him!"

Chapter 21
Chaos Ensues

Samantha woke up full of beans ... aside from the dull throb behind her eyes that reminded her that red wine and spring rolls are a deceptively lethal combo. Nothing an electrolyte sachet and a face dunk in basin of cold water wouldn't fix, though.

She stretched out luxuriously, a satisfied smirk tugging at her lips.

In part, it was the anticipation of that "It's been *way* too long, throw me against the wall" kind of reunion sex that Karen had been obsessing over for days.

"It will be so *intense*," she purred. "Go all out. How about a fresh trim? Ooh, you could get a Vietnamese flag! That'll shock him."

Samantha chuckled. "You're a horny cow, Karen."

But it wasn't just about Kev.

It was about the business.

Lorena's return to SOS would allow Samantha to step into a more strategic role. Give her more time for other ... things.

And with that, she was back to Kev again. The smirk broadened into a smile.

Then ...

BANG!

The door slammed open, hitting the wall with such force that it nearly knocked her out of bed.

James just stood there. Pale. Eyes wide. Chest heaving. "Sammie! Richie's missing."

The words punched the breath right out of her.

Before she could react, James collapsed to the floor, his body racked with primal sobs. "I can't get hold of him," he wailed, clutching at his hair. "He always answers. *Always!* But today, nothing."

Lorena sat bolt upright, the colour draining from her face.

Samantha's heartbeat thundered in her ears, but she forced herself to remain calm. "When did you last speak to him?"

"Last night," James gasped. "He told me he wanted to try again."

Lorena, still groggy, frowned. "Try again? For what?"

"Kids, of course," he screamed, eyes wild. "I told him I wasn't ready. And now he's left me."

Samantha got out of bed, walked across the room, and dropped to her knees beside him. "James, you're not thinking clearly. He wouldn't just leave. You two are ... God, you're *annoyingly* perfect together. Now, what's all this about?"

James hiccupped as he stifled more sobs. "Three years ago, we tried to adopt a baby girl from Vietnam. Everything seemed to be going according to plan, right up to the moment when we transferred the adoption fees. After that, we never heard another thing. We were scammed. That's how we know Kev. He tracked down the gang, reported them to the police, and they were eventually arrested and locked up. Of course, there never was a baby girl, though. The whole thing was utterly traumatic. I can't go through it again. Not yet. Nor can Richie, for that matter. It broke him. But I guess me coming over here stirred up something."

Samantha reached for her phone. "Let me try calling him."

James nodded.

One ring. Two. Three …

Click. A rustle. A breath. Then a weak, groggy voice: "Sammie?"

"Richie," shouted Samantha. "Are you okay?"

"Depends on your definition, darling," he croaked. "I'm knackered. Travelling all night will do that to you. And I think we're completely lost. The taxi driver's been circling Hanoi for hours. What's the name of your hotel again?"

Samantha reeled. "Wait. What? You're in Hanoi?"

"Yes, darling," Richie huffed. "Catch up, will you?"

She barely had a chance to pass on the hotel's name and address before James clawed the phone from her hand.

"You absolute dickhead, Richie! I've been worried sick."

Richie ignored the diatribe. "Apparently we're about an hour away," he yawned. "Kev's out cold on the back seat."

"Kev?" James echoed.

"Yeah," Richie replied casually. "He rang after his little chat with Sammie. Said something about 'no regrets' and asked if I fancied joining him for a surprise visit. I thought, why not?"

Samantha and James stared at each other in giddy disbelief.

"See you soon," Richie said, and hung up.

James threw the phone onto Samantha's bed, then grabbed her by the shoulders. "Right. You heard him. You have one hour. Get your ass in the shower and grab a razor. Trust me, you need one."

Samantha snorted. "Cheeky fecker. But, yeah, you're probably right."

Lorena groaned, flopping back into bed. "Wake me up when the circus rolls into town."

Samantha's heart was pounding.

Richie was coming.

Kev was coming.

Hanoi's sensory overload was about to go into overdrive.

Chapter 22
Oh My

Samantha paced up and down the hotel room, her stomach in knots, palms sweaty, despite the air conditioning.

"Well, this is it. The moment of truth," said Karen. "Will it be fireworks? Or will you discover that Kev's got into oat milk, yoga, and beige slacks since you split up?"

"Shut it," Samantha muttered, smoothing her dress for the hundredth time.

James looked up from the tracking app on his phone, which he'd been frantically refreshing for the last half-hour. "What was that?"

"Nothing," she replied, gripping the back of a chair to stop her legs from buckling under her.

James huffed. "God, I'm nervous. What if Richie sees me and suddenly realizes he needs more than me?"

"James, you literally saved my life. You're a hero. Richie won't be trading you in for a different model. He just wants to move on to the next stage of your relationship. He wants to build a life with you."

James exhaled deeply. "Right. Sure. I'm a catch."

Samantha could tell he wasn't convinced. She was just about to give it another go when there was a vigorous knock on the door.

James sprang up like a jack in the box, ran towards the door, and yanked it open.

Richie was unusually dishevelled, with uncombed hair, a five o'clock shadow, and dark shadows beneath his eyes.

None of that was any deterrent to James, though. "Oh my God, you're really here," he screamed, rushing up to his partner and lifting him off the ground in a tight bear hug. "I thought you'd left me, you absolute wanker."

Richie laughed into James's shoulder. "Missed you too, Jem. More than you could possibly know."

As she watched them cling to each other, James muttering a garbled stream of love declarations interspersed with foul-mouthed insults, Samantha felt her chest ache in the very best way.

Then she heard a gentle cough from the doorway.

"Hey, Sam," said Kev nonchalantly as he stepped over the threshold.

She had prepared a million casual, confident, mature greetings. Unfortunately, what came out was: "What the actual feck are you doing here?"

Kev chuckled and closed the door behind him. "Nice to see you, too."

Samantha folded her arms. "Kev, seriously. Hanoi? That's one hell of a city break."

Kev stepped closer. "Yeah, well, I didn't really have an option. You see, I realized something during that phone call."

She raised an eyebrow, trying not to panic.

"I miss you. I've missed you for years."

Before she had a chance to process what he'd said, he cupped her face in his hands and kissed her.

And it was not a polite, friendly kiss, but a kiss that had been years in the making.

She had two choices:

    1. Pull away and demand answers.

    2. Kiss him back like her life depended on it.

She plumped for Option #2.

Kev pulled her closer.

All that tension, longing, and unfinished business exploded like firecrackers.

It was hardly surprising that they didn't hear the wolf whistle.

But then Richie clapped his hands together like an overenthusiastic school mum. "I *told* you. Pay up."

James sighed, reached into his back pocket, pulled out his wallet, and handed over a crisp twenty-pound note.

Kev finally broke off from the kiss to speak. "You *bet* on us?"

Richie shrugged. "Of course. Jem here was banking on at least an hour of restraint, whereas I knew there'd be no stopping you."

Samantha rolled her eyes, then felt Kev's fingers brushing her cheek again.

"Sam," he said. "Can we talk? Properly, I mean."

"I know the perfect spot," she replied. "You got walking shoes?"

"Trainers. Will they do?" Samantha nodded. "Just let me grab a quick shower. Meet you in the lobby in twenty?"

"Deal."

Kev sprinted to his room, while Samantha headed for the hotel café. She bought a selection of sandwiches, her hand trembling with nervous anticipation as she paid the cashier. Then she made her way to the lobby, sat down, and tried to relax. But by now her whole body was shaking.

Kev emerged from the lift bang on time. He looked fresh, casual, confident. "Ready?" he asked.

"Ready," she lied.

They walked side by side to a nearby park. Then she took his hand and led him to a bench under a large banyan tree.

She handed him a sandwich as they sat down. "Figured we'd need some fuel for this." They ate in silence for a few moments, then she took a deep breath. "Kev, I've been thinking about us. About what happened. I was so focused on work, I left you behind. I'm sorry."

Kev just nodded, his eyes steady.

"I didn't want to fail SOS. Didn't want to fail my dad. But in the end, I failed us, because I ran away. And, if I'm honest, I've been running ever since. But now … I'm ready to stop running."

Kev laced his fingers through hers. "No more running," he said quietly. "Let's face life together. Whatever it looks like. From the moment I saw you that day in the café, I knew I should have fought harder for us. We were great together, Sam. We can be again."

She gripped his hand tightly as he leaned in to kiss her, gently this time.

"So," he whispered. "What now? A couple of laps around the park? Get those steps in?"

She laughed. "You know me too well."

They stood, hand in hand.

All Samantha's anxiety had disappeared. In its place, hope.

Chapter 23

Learning to Say Goodbye

James and Richie chorused, "Ah, isn't young love wonderful," when Kev insisted on making sure that Samantha got home safely.

"Jealous," she said. But then she gave them both a big hug and told James their early-morning walks would be resuming soon. "Maybe not tomorrow, though," she added, with a salacious glance towards Kev.

However, by the time they arrived at her place, the rigours of intercontinental travel were starting to take their toll. Rather than running straight to the bedroom, they curled up on the sofa, each with a cup of tea. Kev reached for a coaster, but inadvertently grabbed hold of an envelope that was sitting on the side table.

"What's this?" he asked, handing it to her.

Samantha recognized it immediately: the eulogy she'd written and recited at her mother's funeral. She hadn't opened the envelope since that day. Her fingers hovered over the flap, tracing the edge for half a minute before she finally reached inside and extracted two sheets of writing paper. Her eyes welled with tears as she stared blankly at her own handwriting.

"Would you read it for me? Aloud?" she whispered.

"Of course," said Kev, confused until he took the pages from her and realized what he was holding. His voice was calm and clear at first, but faltered as the words struck deeper.

> Today, we gather here to remember my beloved mother, Carmel, and to celebrate her life.
>
> Words like "gentle soul", "dignified", "cheerful", and "kind" have been used many times over the past few weeks to describe Mum. These words are all true. We are immensely proud that she was ours.
>
> She was a remarkable, resilient, and resourceful woman with a deep faith in God. She loved her family profoundly and gave her time generously, supporting the youth club, the Scouts, and most recently volunteering at the community centre, which she jokingly referred to as the "old folks' centre", even though, at seventy, she certainly didn't see herself as old.
>
> Mum began working at the age of just fourteen. It was the first demonstration of a

strong work ethic that she carried throughout her life. Sometimes she worked two jobs; sometimes she ran her own businesses. She walked miles to and from work and never once complained. She was bright, capable, and humble.

Samantha snuggled up to Kev, worming her way under his arm to rest her head on his chest, silent tears slipping down her cheeks. She didn't wipe them away. She didn't try to stop them. For the first time, she allowed herself to feel everything – the grief, the love, the loss.

Kev continued reading:

Mum adored children. She was a natural teacher, truly in her element running the playschool, where she nurtured hundreds of kids' curiosity and independence.

She was my rock, always there when I needed her. She had a presence that could stop you in your tracks with a single look. Though fiercely independent herself, she was always grateful for the kindness of those around her. She leaned on her friends but never let it diminish her sense of pride.

Our family holidays were chaotic but joyful, almost always interrupted by some bizarre weather event. Hurricanes. Floods. Ice storms in July. And yet, regardless of what the climate threw at us, she'd insist on a group dip in the freezing North Atlantic until our lips turned blue.

She found her spark again in her seventieth year, travelling to Ireland, Spain, the Aran Islands, and Italy, laughing more, living lighter. Almost as if she knew it would be her last chance.

Mum, my best friend, never wanted to lose her independence or, as she called it, "get alltimers". Over the years, she developed her own unique vocabulary, what we affectionately called "Carmelisms".

She lived life on her own terms. And if she could have chosen a way to leave this world, it would've been as simple as someone switching off a light.

In the end, she got her wish.

Kev paused and looked down at Samantha's flushed, tear-streaked face. Then he read the poem she had chosen for her mum:

When tomorrow starts without me,
Please try to understand,

> That an angel came and called my name,
> And took me by the hand.

His voice broke halfway through the final line. He placed the two sheets of paper back in the envelope and enveloped Samantha, pulling her even closer.

"You okay?" he asked quietly.

She nodded against his shirt. "Yeah."

They sat there in silence, letting the moment settle. But it wasn't a heavy silence. There was no regret, guilt, or words left unsaid.

It was still.

Complete.

Healing.

Finally, Kev stroked her hair and said, "You know, given that she loved children so much, we really should practise making some."

Samantha let out a snort of snotty laughter through her tears, shaking her head. "My mother got everything she ever wanted, but she might have to wait a little longer for a grandchild."

"Technically, that's not a no."

She looked up at him, her eyes still glistening but brighter now. "That's not a no."

"Thank God for that," he whispered.

Samantha suddenly began to hum, then softly sing: "Let it go … let it go …"

Kev raised an eyebrow, bemused. "*Frozen*? Really?"

"Closure," she said, sighing deeply. "Finally. Closure."

One chapter had ended … so a new one could begin.

Donna Abel

Chapter 24

Baby Love

Samantha was deep in the middle of a typically infuriating phone call with IT, demanding to know why her laptop had frozen for the third time that week. Then

Bam!

Her office door burst open in a hurricane of colour, glitter, and unrestrained elation. A squad of cheerleaders stormed in, all pompoms, high kicks, and megawatt grins.

Before Samantha could ask what the hell was happening, the group broke into a choreographed chant that shook the walls:

It's Richie and James's baby time!

Nappies, bottles, cuddles too!

They want it all

Even the poo!

Keep the date

Twentieth of June

You'll meet the baby

Get ready to swoon!

With that, they cartwheeled out of the door.

Samantha and Lorena stared at each other, mouths wide open in silent shock.

"Oh my God!" squealed Samantha, jumping up and down like a giddy teenager. "It's finally happened. The adoption must have gone through." She immediately disconnected the call to the bemused IT department and phoned Richie. "Oh my God!" she shrieked again. "That was the most *you* invitation I've ever received. Congratulations!"

Richie's joy vibrated through the phone. "Thank you, darling. Now, calm down and listen. We've been a bit busy, as you can imagine, so we only had time to come up with one invitation chant for everyone. But we'd love it if you could stop by tonight. We want to ask you something before the christening."

"I'm already in the car," Samantha said, grabbing her bag.

"James wants coffee," Richie added.

"Flat white with oat milk – got it," she said.

"I love you," James shouted in the background.

***

Coffee in hand, Samantha all but sprinted to Richie and James's front door. It swung open before she had a chance to knock.

And there they were: Richie, James … and the most heart-melting little bundle of perfection Samantha had ever seen.

"Meet our daughter," said Richie, glowing with pride. "This is Joy. Say hello, Sammie."

James stepped forward, cradling the tiny child with due reverence.

"Hello, Joy," said Samantha. "I hope you realize you're the luckiest little girl in the world."

"We're hoping she might get a bit luckier," said James, sharing a glance with Richie. "We wondered if you might agree to be her godmother?"

Samantha was still staring in awe at the baby, so it was a couple of moments before she registered what James had said. Only then did she gasp, "Are you serious?"

The two fathers nodded in unison.

"Of course!" she cried, utterly overwhelmed. "It would be the biggest honour of my life."

Joy blinked up at her with wide, curious eyes, hiccupped, then let out such a tiny, adorable sneeze that Samantha almost dissolved on the spot.

"I will protect this child with my life," she declared emphatically.

Richie grinned. "That's exactly what we were hoping for."

Samantha traced a fingertip down Joy's soft cheek. "Did you hear that, Joy? I'm your fairy godmother. You can call me Sammie G."

James burst out laughing. "Sammie G? That's going on the christening invitations."

Inside, a bottle of champagne and three glasses were already laid out on the living-room table.

"To Baby Joy," said Richie, lifting his glass, eyes shining. "May the world be kind to you … and may you sleep through the night!"

"To Joy!" James and Samantha echoed, glasses clinking, hearts full to bursting.

They spent the next few hours staring at her, taking turns to hold her, cherishing her newness. The air felt sacred – like the universe had paused just for them.

**

Then Kev arrived … and instantly lost all his familiar self-composure.

He trembled when Joy was placed in his arms, then started rocking her gently, whispering sweet nothings in her ear.

As she watched them together, Samantha's chest ached with something warm and slow and certain.

It had been months since she'd last heard from Karen, but this was her cue to make a sudden, unexpected reappearance. "Joy's going to need a playmate," she suggested.

Samantha couldn't helping smiling at the idea.

Kev looked over to her, as if he could read her mind, and carefully handed the baby back to James. Then, without warning, he turned to Samantha, dropped to one knee, pulled a small velvet box from his pocket, and opened the lid to reveal the most exquisite princess-cut diamond she'd ever seen.

"Samantha O'Sullivan … will you marry me?"

James and Richie exchanged anxious, expectant glances. Even Baby Joy seemed to hold her breath.

Tears welled in Samantha's eyes as she looked down at the man who had waited for her. Then she whispered, "Yes. A million times, yes."

James and Richie exploded in celebration.

There were cheers, laughter, spilt champagne, and, from Joy, the most perfectly timed giggle in human history.

"Told you," said Richie. "Pay up."

"Every bloody time," grumbled James, handing over another twenty. "Best twenty quid I ever lost, though," he said, raising a glass to Samantha and Kev.

At that precise moment, Samantha realized this was all she'd ever needed.

Family. Love. Joy.

But the story wasn't ending. It was just beginning.

Then Karen asked, "Did you ever get the results of that menopause test?"

Ah feck off...

My Journal
The Secret Diary of a Trek Virgin

<u>Entry 1 – The Morning After the Night Before</u>

Ahh, no. What the feck did I do? Shit, shit, shit. Feckin' hell. Vietnam? What was I thinking?

But worse than that ... the shame. Did I really yell "Winner, winner, chicken dinner" in front of a room full of people? Where did that even come from? What a total loser.

Oh, my head. My poor head. Why did I choose last night to drink so much? I haven't touched alcohol since Mum's funeral, so why now? Shame on me for having fun.

But God, I did love the dancing. It reminded me of family weddings when you just let go and stomp around the dance floor like you own it. I've not done that in years.

Note to self: Must get fitter. Sweating like a hostage mid-dance is not a good look.

My pure, undiluted hatred for the Lousy Dosser remains as strong as ever. Why would she bid against me at a charity auction, for feck's sake? Isn't it enough that she steals my best clients- bitch.

And to think I rated her. She had talent, potential, and a sharp business brain. All that was lacking was patience. But she's been a total bitch since she left SOS.

Right, enough of her. I need to find out more about this trip. Surely, it can't be that challenging, can it? It's a charity trek, not the bloody SAS.

God, I hope it's easy. Because I have zero time for training.

Entry 2 – Not So Happy Paddy's Day

I felt very lonely today. Missing Mum.

She loved Paddy's Day. Always making boiled bacon and cabbage with potatoes. God, I miss that. But not as much as I miss her.

I picked up the phone to call her today. It wasn't until I was holding it in my hand that I realized what I was doing. Jesus, I must be losing my mind.

Why would I do that? I'm feeling like such a loser.

Of course, thoughts of Mum often lead to thoughts of Kev. They were so close, even after we split up. Today, for the first time in years, I seriously considered sending him a text, but then thought better of it. I guess the past should stay in the past.

Trek news: Oh my God, it turns out it's going to be MUCH harder than I hoped.

I finally got round to reading the pack today. The pack I won ... if you can call it winning. Sweet Jesus.

I'm going to have to make time for training, otherwise I might not survive.

I reckon first thing in the morning is the best plan. I love the sunrise. And maybe it'll take my mind off my shitty life. It might even help me get some sleep.

I'm DESPERATE for a good night's sleep. A night when I don't:

- *Wake up sweating.*
- *Have nightmares that we buried Mum alive.*

Right! Stop feeling sorry for yourself and get ready for training.

Entry 3 – Yay, I've Finally Started

Training has begun. And by training, I mean I went for a swim. Which counts. I think.

Because, if walking is good training, surely swimming is better? Less pressure on the joints, full-body workout, chance of drowning if you don't keep moving ... all that jazz.

But instead of feeling strong and accomplished, I am currently experiencing the burning humiliation of being overtaken in a swimming pool by a woman who was WALKING.

Feckin' WALKING. Not only that – she bloody lapped me ... four times. ON FOOT.

And the cheeky mare put her towel right next to mine, even though there were loads of empty loungers. It really pissed me off. I was in such a rage I could have scratched her eyes out.

Why am I so angry all the time? Maybe walking will calm me down.

I feel mentally exhausted and I know that I'm snappy, unapproachable, letting silly stuff get on top of me. Why am I so weak? I used to be so much more resilient than this.

Get a grip, Sammie. It's time to face your future.

Pull up your big girl's pants.

I need to keep going, battle on.

Dear Morpheus, please be kind tonight and let me get some sleep.

<u>Entry 4 – Time Flyies</u>

Can't believe it's still feckin' March. Why is this such a long month?

I decided today was going to be my first training walk. Set the new alarm on my phone for 5:15. It screams, "GET UP, GET UP, GET UP, YOU LAZY ARSE, GET UP NOW!" until you make it stop.

Last night's forecast predicted no rain, but of course it absolutely pissed down, didn't it! I was soaked to the bone, and my body was all blotchy by the time I got home and staggered into the shower. Gross. I felt physically sick at the sight of myself. That's a new low even for me. I'm wondering if I might have contracted pneumonia, too. Probably should see a doctor. But not HER. Not now.

Still seething about the Lousy Dosser. She's competing with us for every contract now, and winning some of them. Got to keep moving and work even harder.

My poor team. It's a good job I'm travelling in the coming weeks. It'll give them a much-needed break from me. We used to walk on sunshine, but now they're walking on eggshells.

Donna Abel

Entry 5 – Why Am I Such a Fool

Feeling utterly overwhelmed. I've been working fourteen-hour days for seven days in a row. Can't be arsed to go out tonight. Who needs to eat anyway? Not me, it seems. The weight's been falling off me. Who knew that having a shitty time would result in so many people telling you you look amazing? Feck off, I'm dying inside!

Oh, here's something new: I've started talking to myself, out loud. I really am losing the plot.

I couldn't wait to leave the office today. Alex is uptight about something, which is affecting his work, and Mary is just plain annoying. She's such a do-gooder that I start snapping at her, then I feel guilty because she's only trying to be nice.

Work is still crazy busy. We really need to land this project, especially after losing the last one to LD. I wonder if the Lousy Dosser knows that she might be doing her former colleagues/friends out of a job. Feeling a massive amount of pressure. I don't want to let anyone go, but there might be no option.

Walked in the sunshine today, which made it easier to clock up the miles, but I need to find a decent walking partner to keep up the momentum.

- *No pricks*

- *No wankers*
- *No dickheads*
- *No princesses*

Feck! A thought just occurred to me. What if I manage to find someone and they think that I'm a prick ... or a dickhead ... or a wanker? Or, worst of all, a princess!

Entry 6 – Killer Steak for Dinner

Met up with Nico tonight. He's like a second dad to me. He gets me, and he makes me feel as if I can do anything. Well, anything work-related. He did laugh a bit too hard when I told him about the trek.

I ate like a horse. Nico insisted on three courses and I'm so glad he did. Dessert was delish.

Now my eyes are feeling heavy, so ...

Night, night x

Had an amazing two hours of sleep – the best for years – but woke up in a massive amount of pain. My stomach is killing me. Maybe I have an ulcer? Or worse? That reminds me, I must get my will in order. So many people depend on me. I need to catch this life-threatening illness early or I might not survive.

Do I want to survive?

Yes, I do. But only if I can get back to how I used to be, without a hit squad of inner demons constantly bullying me.

Can't put it off any longer. I'll make an appointment with Dr Heartless tomorrow.

Entry 7 – The Willy Kink

What on earth was I thinking, placing that advert in the paper. How seedy did it sound? I'm surprised they even printed it. Good job I didn't put my real name to it.

Jesus, I've never seen so many willies!

I showed Jo and Laura some of the more interesting specimens. Laura was convinced she recognized one of them. It had a piercing and what she called "a bit of a weird kink". Apparently, the guy called it Shmoopy!

We laughed till we cried, but I'm no closer to finding a walking partner.

Oh well, I guess I'll just have to join the dreaded walking group. Maybe one of them will want to get in some extra practice before breakfast? If not, I might need to make my excuses and drop out. So far, I think the best idea is to wander close to a cliff edge and fake an attack of vertigo.

I made the appointment to see the quack. Can't wait!

Entry 8 – Walking Woes

I practised some new walking styles today. Yes, really! They're all feckin' shocking. How the hell can I do a trek when I can't even walk properly?

To cheer myself up, I jumped head first into some serious retail therapy. Amazingly, it turns out that shopping for walking gear is a lot of fun. It's an amazing new world of laceless boots, Gore-Tex, anti-chafe fabrics, breathable mid-layers (whatever the feck they are), and fluorescent colours. Spent a small fortune but at least I'll look the part now ... if I can figure out how to put one foot in front of the other without looking like a drunken giraffe.

Entry 9 – How Bloody Rude

That doctor really bloody hates me. She practically threw me out of the consulting room. What did I ever do to her? I could tell she was trying not to laugh when I asked her to check me for DVT. How can she be so sure that's not the cause of my aching legs? I Googled it and found a report that said lack of sleep could lead to DVT. Well, I'm lucky to get three hours' sleep a night! As for the night sweats ... she was just as dismissive of my suggestion that it might be a symptom of early-onset menopause. I really need to find a new GP. One who's not such a cow.

Meanwhile, we've all been slaving over the pitch. We need this contract so much, but it feels like the Lousy Dosser is always one step ahead of us.

Officially well and truly fed up!

Entry 10 – Teary Eyed ... Twice

Well, I did the dreaded group walk today ... and survived! All I wanted to do when I got home was call Mum and tell her all about it. Had a little weep when I remembered I can't do that any more.

Eloise is great. She listened without judging while I shared my views about Dr Heartless. Then she dropped the bombshell that she not only knows her from previous treks but that she's her sister-in-law! FFS, I really should engage my brain before shouting my mouth off.

It was a relief to learn that the not-so-good doctor won't be accompanying us to Vietnam, but harder to hear that the reason for her absence is that she thinks I'm a narcissist. That really hurts. In fact, I'm crying again just thinking about it. I could cope with being called a princess, but a narcissist? That's just not right.

On a more positive note, Walk #2 seems to be working for me. Not so much leg pain today, so I'm willing to concede that Dr Heartless MIGHT have been right when she said I haven't got DVT. Still think I might be menopausal, though.

The new walking gear attracted some admiring glances from the rest of the group. Or maybe they were smirking because I'd forgotten to remove the tags. One of the guys pulled them off and handed them to me. Cheeky bastard ... but he seems friendly.

Google fact of the day: Apparently walking is good for your mood.

Fingers crossed THAT proves to be true.

Entry 11 – Feeling Good

Actually had a good night's sleep. Wonders will never cease!

I've been thinking about Kev for some reason. I wonder what he's doing. Wonder if he's even still in Jersey. I blame Adele's song "Hello" for this – I heard it twice today. But let's get real, he probably wouldn't want to hear from me. He's probably moved on. Maybe *the past is better left in the past, and all those memories should stay there. I wish I'd ended it better, but it's done now. Can't change it. Have to live with it.*

Anyway, onwards and upwards!

Tomorrow we'll put the finishing touches to the pitch. It's been such hard work – for me more than anyone – but I'm so proud of what we've achieved. Feeling positive.

Entry 12 – Thanatophobia

Learned a new word today. Thanatophobia – the fear of losing someone you love.

Sometimes I hate small talk, sometimes it's better NOT to talk. Today Mary informed me that, on average, people fall in love seven times before they get married. I'm not sure why she shared this little nugget with me.

I honestly think I've got a six-year emotional hangover from Kev. Maybe I still ... NO! Let's not go there.

I'm excited about the pitch. It's almost done. Just need Alex to work his magic and give it that final polish.

Sent a WhatsApp to the walking group. No replies, but with a bit of luck someone will show up for an early walk tomorrow.

Off to bed, now. Hoping for three good nights' sleep in a row.

Entry 13 – The Shame

Oh my good God! WTAF!

How will I ever get over it? I'm totally mortified. My guts just exploded on the cliff path. Even writing about it is making me cringe. I wanted the ground to open up and swallow me whole. Thank feck the only person to witness it was James – the guy from the hiking group who pulled off my price tags. He's a keeper. I'm sure we'll laugh about it in the future ... WAY in the future, in my case.

For now, the shame is still burning far too bright. As is the pain, for that matter. My side is killing me. I guess I must have pulled a muscle. I'm going to grab an ice pack, take a bucketload of painkillers, and go straight to bed, because I feel like shit.

No pun intended.

Entry 14 – May the Force Be with You

Well, it's been a while. Did you miss me?

Apparently, I could have died. I've had more than a few encounters with old Dr Heartless over the last few days. It seems I may have misjudged her. She was genuinely bemused when I told her I knew she'd called me a narcissist. But if it's not me, who the hell is it?

It was great to see the team when they visited. Alex worked day and night to put the finishing touches to the pitch, then submitted it on my behalf. And Cris was so kind to go to my place and fetch this journal for me.

The hospital isn't so bad. It's nice to relax for a bit and have my meals cooked and bed changed. The drugs are ... interesting, too. I've never felt so giddy and giggly in my life! Some of the other side effects are less enjoyable, though. I had a weird dream—or more like a nightmare—that the Lousy Dosser was going on the trek. Hope it doesn't prove to be a recurring one!

Entry 15 – Old Enemies and New Friends

It wasn't a dream! The Lousy Dosser is really coming to Vietnam! So I guess we now know the identity of the narcissistic princess. But I need to forget about her and concentrate on my recovery, my work, and my friends. Taking of which ...

I've met the most incredible person – James's partner, Richie. He's so full of infectious energy and over-the-top enthusiasm. Although I would not recommend laughing with an appendix scar and twelve stitches! He and James are the sweetest couple – so caring. It'll be impossible to fall into a funk with them around.

Slept six hours. Whoop!

Entry 16 – Feeling Uneasy

I think I may have overdone it. I was feeling great last week, but this week my emotions are like a rollercoaster. I have a very strange feeling I can't shake – like I'm being watched or even spied on. I'm hoping it's just paranoia – maybe a bizarre side-effect of coming off the meds? Either that or I'm being haunted.

Received a lovely message from Tricia – a girl from the walking group who had "a bit of an accident" well she pissed her pants during one of the hikes. As a joke, I sent her a colostomy bag and she replied to tell me she loved it. I think we will get on well. I wonder what she'd send me if she knew about the poonami! Thankfully, James hasn't told a soul about it – not even Richie.

Apparently, we'll hear about the contract next week. Feeling anxious, but confident. It was such a great team effort that I don't see how we can lose.

Entry 17 – Always Trust Your Gut

Fuming! We didn't win the contract. Guess who did?

FFS, how is this possible? How is a one-man band with next to no experience of running her own company able to swoop in and steal such a big contract from right under our noses?

Okay, I know I sound like a sore loser. Like the time when we were playing musical chairs and Mum made me sit on the sidelines and watch after I complained that one of the other girls had pushed me. But I was only six! I like to think I've matured a bit since then. If it had been a fair fight, I'd take it on the chin and move on. But something's not right about this. It makes no sense. I need to look into it.

Plan for tomorrow:

1. *Speak to James and Richie and ask for their honest opinion.*
2. *Find out what the feck is going on.*
3. *Try not to spiral.*

Entry 18 – 00Sammie

James and Richie insist it's not paranoia. They think it's sabotage. I agree, but I can't start pointing impatient fingers at everyone and accusing them of industrial espionage. I need to stay calm, composed, and cool if I'm to get to the bottom of this. And a bit of help from a professional wouldn't go amiss.

Fortunately, Richie knows a private detective. (I didn't ask why!) He gave me the guy's contact details, and I've arranged to meet him.

Entry 19 – As Faith Would Have It

What an incredible day. It turns out that Kev – MY Kev (well, not my Kev any more, but you get the point) – is the private investigator. What are the chances?

My poor heart practically exploded when I saw him walk through the door. He hasn't changed a bit – same eyes, same smile, same ability to make my brain short-circuit. I can't help thinking that Mum is orchestrating the whole thing from up above, like some celestial matchmaker. She always loved a good romance. Not to mention bad ones. I nearly died of embarrassment when she asked to borrow my copy of Fifty Shades of

Grey. My face heats up like a radiator just thinking about her reading it and wondering if I was into all that stuff.

Back to the present, though. Kev is back in my life, and I'm freaking out about it. A tsunami of guilt is crashing over me for walking out on him, for choosing my job over the future that could have been ours. But I've got to remain detached. This is strictly business, transactional even. Nothing more. We met because I'm paying him to do a job, not to rekindle anything. Professional – that's us.

Then again ... I can't help wondering if he's spent the last six years thinking about me. Asking, "What if?"

I'm so screwed.

Entry 20 – Rat-Catching

There's a rat in my business, what am I going to do? Fix that rat, that's what I'm going to do.

That song will be in my head all night now. I used to love watching Mum jump around the kitchen whenever it came on the radio. (She hated rats, God bless her.)

I've just Googled it. Apparently, the lyrics refer to Maggie Thatcher. Dad would've loved that bit of trivia. But he'd be furious that someone is hurting not just me but my business and my employees. And for what? That's the key question. Why would someone do this? What do they stand to gain? Or is it just a spiteful fucker who wants to ruin me?

Kev asked me to draw up a strategy while he pores over the data.

Here's my draft checklist:

Look for people with influence in the company:
- *Include those I least suspect. (Note to self: Trust no one. Paranoia is your new friend.)*
- *Total number of rats? One? Two? An entire nest? (Jesus, I hope not!)*

Identify possible entry points:
- *IT systems.*
- *Boardroom leaks.*
- *New employees and interns who seem too good to be true.*

Prepare the "Rat Control Treatment" (Kev's term):
- *Bait the trap with some juicy, misleading information and see who bites.*

Block entry points and remove access:
- *Change passwords ... again.*

- *Shred all sticky notes at the end of the day.*

Thoroughly sanitize the workforce:
- *Not literally. (With the possible exception of Jax. What is it about teenagers and hygiene?)*
- *Hold a team meeting to remind everyone that I see all, hear all, and have caffeine-fuelled omniscience.*

Kev read the list and smiled. He said it reminded him of playing cards with my mother. I'd completely forgotten that we swapped her cards whenever she went to the loo. Sometimes a bit of deviousness can work wonders.

Entry 21 – The List of the Pissed!

I've been trying to compile a list of everyone who might have a reason to betray me. Unfortunately, I haven't got very far. The only name on it is Mary's ... and even that's a long shot. Maybe she thought I was having a dig at her when I told her I was too young for menopause? But it wasn't as if I gave her a gift card for a course of Botox! As for the rest of the team ... they've all been so supportive since Mum's death. I hate the idea of suspecting any of them.

So it looks like it's down to Kev. Here's hoping he'll uncover the identity of whoever's leaking information to the Lousy Dosser. Otherwise, I'm doomed.

Dear Morpheus

Please sprinkle some sleep dust on me tonight. I've got a busy day tomorrow. Business as usual, Chamber of Commerce lunch, and must try to squeeze in a few miles for the trek.

Really, really need to get some sleep.

Night night x

Entry 22 – Cat and Mouse to Catch a Rat

I'm obsessing about catching the rat. Kev told me the trap's been set, the bait's been laid, now we just need to wait for someone to bite. Fingers and toes crossed. I feel sick with nerves and paranoia, like my stomach is permanently clenched in a tight fist. I long to get back to walking, put all this suffocating dread behind me, feel the ground under my feet and the fresh air in my lungs, ideally with James by my side.

Kev is still convinced that the culprit must be a member of my leadership team, as no one else had access to the data that was leaked to the Lousy Dosser. I just can't see it, though. Or rather, I don't want to see it. That level of betrayal would be a massive stab in the back. But I have to know the truth.

Please take the bait, you horrible rat, and get out of my life for ever.

But then what? What happens when it's over? When the rat is exposed and Kev walks out of my life again.

I thought I was handling it well – keeping it professional and businesslike. But I feel my resolve crumbling away every time Kev looks at me with those eyes. I catch myself daydreaming about the way he moves, the way he smiles, the way his voice softens when he talks to me, his smell. It's so pathetic. I'm pathetic.

The worst part is that he IS being entirely professional. There are no lingering touches, no meaningful looks. It's just business for him. I guess that's a good thing. After all, this will soon be over. Then we can have a clean break. Rip the plaster off. No point dwelling on what might have been or what will never be.

And yet ... my heart aches at the thought of not seeing him again. Of him walking out of my life – for good this time.

I can't believe I'm saying this, but maybe it wouldn't be so bad if the rat continued to run free for another week. At least that would give me another seven days to be near Kev, hear his voice, see his smile. Another seven days before I have to say goodbye again.

I keep replaying it all in my head: the last time we spoke before I walked out on him; his stunned expression, like he couldn't believe I was leaving. I never really apologised, not properly. I didn't have the words.

I wish I could turn back time. I wish I hadn't chosen job, ambition, the endless bloody cycle of work over him. Over us. But it's too late now. Made my bed, blah, blah, blah ...

So, I'll just focus on the rat. It's simpler that way. Anger is simpler. Betrayal is simpler. If I start picking at the wounds left by Kev, I don't think I'll be able to stop.

God, I need to sleep. Everything changes tomorrow, one way or another.

Night night x

Entry 23 – Kev Was Right!

Gutted! It was Alex!

I had no clue, none whatsoever, but he was caught red-handed. The cheeky git told me he'd see me in court. No remorse. No apology.

Hayden was fabulous. She had my back. Her tone was perfect – calm, measured, but pointed. Even I found her a bit scary. I don't think there'll be a tribunal.

God, I loved playing Lord Sugar. "You're fired!" What a badass I am.

It gave me a massive surge of adrenaline, but then, strangely, there was no relief, no joy. Instead, I felt completely empty.

After consulting Dr Google, I learned that the mind can shut down feelings in order to protect itself in periods of heightened emotion. It's a bit like your brain saying, "This is a lot to deal with right now, so let's take a break and come back to it later."

My other doctor – the real one – has advised me to take a few weeks off. She reckons I'm emotionally burned out. I think she's probably right. I'll work half days for the next three weeks and get in some much-needed walking practice. Then I'll try not to think about work from the moment I board the plane to Vietnam to the day I get back.

Entry 24 – Life Goes On

> Dear Dad,
> Happy Heavenly Birthday!
> I miss you. I hope you're proud of SOS. Have a whiskey on me.
> I received lots of messages today from friends and family saying, "Cherish the memories, and remember he's always with you." I do hope so.
> I also hope that you and Mum are having a whale of a time – reunited and keeping a close eye on everything.
> Until we meet again … love you always and for ever.
> Sammie xoxo

The rat saga was just a bump in the road. It's over now, so I can move forward – "Just keep swimming," as Richie constantly reminds me.

Vietnam's coming at the perfect time. It'll enable me to draw a line under the last few months. Then things will be different when I get back.

Checklist for post-Vietnam life:
- *Live a little. There's nothing wrong with a bit of drama. Bring on the chaos!*
- *Take holidays*
- *Make time for friends who ask, "How are you?" and actually want to hear the answer*
- *Keep walking*
- *Work no more than a forty-hour week*
- *Take weekends off*
- *Continue to support the charity*
- *Find a man to love (or take a chance with one you've already found)*
- *Don't hold grudges*
- *Stop trying to prove to Dad that you're good enough. He already knows I'm good enough. I just need to believe it myself*
- *Stop listening to Karen*
- *Tell James I'm Katie Green*

Karen was very vocal after Mum died, and she's scarcely shut up since. I guess she was my way of coping. But I think I've found better ways now. Journaling certainly seems to be working for me. Who knew that writing down your innermost thoughts could be so cathartic? (Karen's saying, "Everyone aside from you, you tosser!")

Entry 25 – What Do You Do with Time

Today I realized I've got a lot of time on my hands. It feels odd. What on earth do other people do with it? First I tried to perfect my coffee-making skills. Not bad, but my flat white still needs work. Then I attempted to suck the chocolate off a whole bag of Maltesers without damaging the little biscuit spheres, but my tongue started to feel like sandpaper after fifteen or so. Next, I power-washed the decking. It looks amazing, and it felt good to put in some hard physical graft, but it's hardly a long-term solution to the question of how to fill my days. It'll probably be another five years before it needs doing again.

Time is lucky. It's infinite. It doesn't age or tire. It's consistent ... and a healer, or so they say. I guess they're right about that – whoever "they" are. My latest blister healed in three days. That's quick, right?

Entry 26 – The Art of Sleeping

I've discovered that doing not very much is exhausting. I feel jaded. My eyes are closing as I write this. I even fell asleep watching Jack Reacher (my favourite guilty pleasure). This is unheard of. It seems that even Tom Cruise is incapable of keeping me awake these days.

I've been trying to master the art of sleeping, but it's a losing battle. I've read all the tips: no screens for an hour before bedtime; a cup of chamomile tea (yeuch!); a good book. Nothing seems to work. Maybe I should take up meditation or yoga. Or perhaps I just need a break from everything.

I met James for lunch. I've known him for months now, but it was only today that I learned he's a bigshot lawyer. He's got a lot going on, but can't talk about any of it. It was like having lunch with a secret agent. He's got this air of mystery about him, and I can't help but be intrigued. He's charming, witty, and has a way of making me feel like the most important person in the room. Richie is so lucky to have him. Although, to be honest, James is lucky to have Richie, too. They're perfect together.

James says I'm a good distraction for him. Maybe I'm HIS guilty pleasure. It's nice to know that I provide some relief from his high-stakes world. We talked about everything and nothing. It was so refreshing. I'm really looking forward to the trek, although I wish Richie were come along, too. We'd have such fun together.

Entry 27 – Packing: Two Weeks to Go

I almost forgot to get my jabs! Called Dr Heart in a mad panic, but she said I should be okay as long as I get them today. So, it was straight down to Boots.

Felt like I'd been punched in the arm by the time I got home, so I distracted myself by compiling a list of essentials to pack:

- Lightweight, breathable clothing
- Layers
- Rain gear
- Comfortable hiking boots
- Crocks
- Socks
- Hat
- Sunglasses
- PJs
- Evening clothing
- Celebration night clothing
- Flight clothing

- *Backpack*
- *Water bottle and hydration system*
- *Trekking poles*
- *Sleeping bag and liner*
- *First-aid kit (×2 just in case)*
- *Multitool*
- *Headlamp (aka dickhead light)*
- *Insect repellent*
- *Sunscreen*
- *Snacks*
- *Cash (pounds, dollars, – love it! – dongs)*
- *Bog roll*
- *Poo bags*
- *Shower gel*
- *Dry shampoo*
- *Lip balm*
- *Mascara*
- *Toiletries*
- *Phone*
- *Phone charger*
- *Dry bags*
- *Painkillers*
- *Earplugs*

That should do it!

Note to self: Bog roll should be top of the list!

Entry 28 – Chicken Terror

Supplementary item for the list: tranquillizer gun!

I was strolling through Jersey's rural lanes today, minding my own business, when suddenly a gang of chickens (I refuse to call them a flock – that's far too nice a word for these nutters) decided to launch an all-out attack against me. I swear they were possessed. Their eyes were wild, feathers ruffled, and they were clucking like maniacs. Before I knew it, they were charging at me like a scene from a Hitchcock movie. I don't know if they were defending their territory or just having a bad day. Either way, it was bloody terrifying. I barely escaped with my life.

Okay, maybe I'm being a tad overdramatic, but I've heard there are a lot of chickens in Vietnam, and you can't be too careful, so I plan to be armed.

Entry 29 – Packed and Excited

I feel like a kid who's about to go on a school trip. Two sleeps to go! Whoop, whoop! The excitement is real. My mind and body are tingling at the thought of the adventure ahead, the change of scenery, the newness of it all. I can't wait.

Packing has been an experience in itself. I started with the essentials – ticking off every item the list – but of course I've added a few extras. (No tranquillizer gun, unfortunately. They're surprisingly hard to buy on Amazon.) However, the bag is ridiculously heavy now, so I might need to rethink a few things. Do I really need a travel iron? A backup laptop? A hairdryer? And let's be honest, lugging around a pillow and bath sheets seems like overkill.

I keep telling myself I should be more pragmatic, but there's always that little voice whispering, "What if you need ...?"

One thing I definitely will need? Wet wipes. I packed plenty, so I'll have more than enough to share. Funny how small things like that suddenly become essential. I used to be so careless about packing – just shoving everything into a bag at the last minute. But now ... packing cubes are my best friends. Everything has its place. I like the order, the calm it brings. Oh dear, what have I become?

I've been thinking about the roommate situation. Fingers crossed I'm paired with someone decent. Please, universe, don't let it be the Lousy Dosser. Surely

Eloise wouldn't do that to me, would she? She knows exactly what I think of Lorena, and what the Lousy Dosser thinks of me.

Oh my God, there's a thought. Have I ever told her that we hate each other? We've discussed Dr Heart at great length, but maybe Lorena's never cropped up?

Must stop panicking. It might not happen. And even if it does, I'm sure I can handle it. I've grown, right? I've learned how to deal with difficult people.

Deep breath. I'm sure it'll be fine.

Entry 30 – A Tiny Panic Attack

I can't stop thinking about Kev. It's getting ridiculous. I've even done the social media deep dive – full-blown detective mode. Good news: no recent photos of him looking disgustingly happy with a stunning girlfriend. Could there still be a tiny glimmer of hope?

I almost called him today. Had it all worked out: "How about that raincheck drink? Or dinner? My shout as a thank-you for trapping the rat." But of course I chickened out. I just stared at his name on the screen like a total muppet before throwing the phone onto the bed as if it had personally betrayed me.

Maybe I'll summon up the courage after Vietnam? It'll be easier then. I'll have lots of cool stories to tell him. I might even give him the impression I've transformed myself into a free-spirited, adventurous, effortlessly chill trekker babe. Someone who doesn't stalk her ex's socials at one in the morning while eating cereal straight from the box.

Shit! Do I need a visa for Vietnam? Come on Google, hurry up!

Nope, I'm good. Phew. Crisis, what crisis?

Now, where's that cereal?

Entry 31 – One More Sleep

I've just spent the last three hours looking for my passport. I knew it wasn't LOST lost. I put my cash in it when I was packing. But I was still like a woman possessed – screaming, bawling, throwing cushions around the room. For the life of me, I couldn't remember where I'd put it.

Three bloody hours! And guess where it was. Guess where I'd put it. Yes, in the most logical place imaginable – the secret zip pocket in my backpack.

Note to self: Always make a note of where you've put your bloody passport, you feckin' idiot. (But then does that mean you also need to make a note of where you've left the note? Oh Jesus.)

Showered, shaved, and ready to go. Should I bother packing a razor? It wasn't on the list, but I may as well. There's a bit of room now that I'm not taking the tranquillizer gun.

Excited! One more sleep. If I manage to get any, that is.

Entry 32 – Hanoi

The day has finally arrived! After a night of tossing and turning, I woke up feeling like a kid on Christmas morning. My bags are packed (minus travel iron and hairdryer, plus razor), and I'm ready to embark on this adventure.

The airport was a madhouse. Thousands of people rushing around like headless chickens. I managed to navigate a path through the chaos and even had time for a quick coffee before boarding. Maybe a caffeine hit wasn't the best idea, though, because my mind was racing when we took off.

What if I've forgotten something crucial? What if my roommate is the Lousy Dosser? What if those crazy chickens have cousins in Vietnam?

The flight was long but uneventful. I tried to sleep but ended up watching three movies back-to-back instead. So I felt like a zombie by the time we landed – thoroughly jetlagged and slightly delirious.

Then we stepped off the plane and the heat hit us like a cannonball. Welcome to Hanoi, puny Westerners! Thankfully, the hotel has air-con. It's also charming, with friendly staff and large, comfortable rooms. Dinner was a feast of delicious local delicacies – pho, spring rolls, fresh fruit. We all chatted excitedly about the trek, sharing stories and laughter.

After dinner, James and I took a stroll around the neighbourhood. It was past 10 p.m. but the streets were still buzzing – vendors selling their wares, children playing, motorbikes zipping by at breakneck speed. It was so vibrant and alive – a stark contrast to the quiet lanes of Jersey.

But all that excitement seems a distant memory now that I'm back in my room ... or rather, OUR room. Because, inevitably, I've got a roommate. And, even more inevitably, it's the Lousy Dosser.

Entry 33 – Who Ever Said It's Good to Share?

The universe is just cruel. I begged everyone to swap with me, but they all said I was strong enough to take one for the team. Thanks, guys. Really appreciate it.

I'm fuming! She's SO annoying. Who doesn't put the lid on the toothpaste? Or wipe the mirror after taking a shower? And don't get me started on the quiet act. It's like she's trying to win an Oscar for Best Performance in a Silent Movie. She tiptoes around the room, barely making a sound, as if she's scared to disturb me. It's like she's trying to make out that she's the victim and I'm the bully.

But she was the one who left me in the lurch by abandoning SOS. She was the one who ended our friendship without a backward glance. She was the one who persuaded the rat to spy on me. She's the one who's at fault. Not me. She never even said sorry.

Part of me thinks I should let bygones be bygones and forgive her. But I'm not ready. Not yet. She needs to show some remorse. Until then, I'll continue to call her the Lousy Dosser.

And she can count herself lucky I haven't come up with anything worse.

Entry 34 – Talking, for Feck's Sake

Most of us know that some things should stay safely locked in Pandora's box. Unfortunately, Julie doesn't seem to have got that particular memo. Tonight, while we were all sitting around the dinner table, Eloise invited her to share a story. And, well, she took that invitation and ran with it.

"This is a funny one," she began, swaying slightly. (We were all a few beers in.) "The day before we came here, I got home early from work to find my husband in bed with a blowup doll. But not just any blowup doll. It had my face on it!"

Not a giggle. Not a titter. Utter, stunned silence. But she wasn't done yet.

"The doll looked amazing. It had a better body than I've ever had. And there he was, mid-thrust, going at it like a jackhammer. The whole room stank of cheap plastic. I guess that's better than cheap perfume, right? But here's the kicker: he was having more fun with that doll – which he'd dressed in my actual nightshirt – than we'd had in years."

By this point, I'd stopped breathing. We all had.

Julie sighed dramatically and took a swig of her beer. "The bastard got a massive rubber rash on his knob. Serves him right, I reckon."

Desperate glances were exchanged. One or two mouths started to open, then swiftly clamped shut again.

Finally, it fell to Dr Emily, God bless her, to break the silence. She calmly sipped her drink and said, "I have a cream for that."

And that was it. Everyone erupted. I laughed so hard I nearly choked.

The night ended with us all agreeing that what's said in Vietnam stays in Vietnam. I hope that's true … for Julie's husband's sake!

Entry 35 – Apologies Accepted

I got lost yesterday. Really lost. Totally stranded on a mountainside as night was falling. But that wasn't the most dramatic event of the day. Because guess who was with me?

James has been nagging me to be the bigger person, take the high road, and clear the air with Lorena. So, I dropped back from the rest of the group and tried to talk to her. Of course, as expected, she wasn't having any of it. *She just kept plodding along as if I didn't exist. But then we lost sight of the others. It was getting dark, so we had no option but to stop and make camp.*

I think both of us would rather have been anywhere else in the world – with anyone else in the world – but she was really struggling with blisters, and in a rare moment of maturity (or possibly lack of oxygen to the brain) I extended an olive branch. I loaned her a pair of my socks. My favourite socks! The bright yellow ones. I guess I'll never see them again. But you know what? I don't care. Because that little gesture changed EVERYTHING between us. It was like a key was turned and the floodgates opened.

First, she told me that she didn't steal the contract. Of course, I was sceptical, but I must admit that everything she said made perfect sense. It was Alex who was the rat, not Lorena.

Then, she explained that she's doing the trek on behalf of her dad, who's been diagnosed with Parkinson's. I've met him a few times and he's such a great guy. He does not deserve this. How much of a self-centred cow have I been, thinking she signed up just to spite me?

Thankfully, that was when the rest of the group found us.

But the talking didn't end there. Back here at the guest house, it continued for hours. She cried; I cried. She laughed; I laughed. She apologized for leaving SOS; I apologized for assuming she was conducting a personal vendetta against me.

By the end of it all, it was like a weight had lifted off me. I felt like I'd regained a friend. And maybe even a colleague: I'm thinking of asking her to come back to SOS.

I know one conversation won't change the past, but it's given me so much hope for the future.

I can finally move on and think about ... Well, let's be honest, KEV.

I just can't get him out of my head.

Now, though, I really need to get some sleep. The trek resumes in two hours!

<u>Entry 36 – The Final Stretch</u>

I didn't find full enlightenment on a mountaintop. There was no cinematic sunrise moment when the wind whispered closely guarded secrets. No slow-motion montage with a Coldplay soundtrack.

Instead, I was a complete mess – crying like a baby, moaning like a bitch, just wanting to get it done. I was exhausted and it was bloody hard work.

But I did get a bit of closure. There was a moment when I was sure I had reconnected with Mum. It gave me a chance to say goodbye. I hope I've made her proud.

I wish Richie had been there to greet us with his pompoms, shouting chants of encouragement, but James was great. Calm and positive, always armed with blister plasters and a kick up the ass when I needed it.

Still thinking of Kev. I've decided to give him a call when we get back.

In the meantime, it's the celebration meal tonight. Can't wait! But I must remember not to drink too much. We've all seen the consequences of that, haven't we, Julie!

Entry 37 – Drunk Dialling

The celebration dinner was fantastic. I had such a great time – laughing, dancing, hugging people who were little more than strangers a week ago. What a way to end the trek!

But I couldn't leave it there, could I? Of course not.

Drunk as a skunk, still riding the emotional high of reaching the summit, I only went and CALLED HIM.

What ... a ... dickhead. I really need to learn some self-control.

It was stupidly late. I barely remember what I said – something about feeling brave and maybe a bit lost and "Please come and find me"?

Oh my God!

Entry 38 – No Turning Back

He came to find me!

Kev is here ... in Hanoi.

I'm writing this with him snoring gently beside me. Can you believe it?

I don't know how to put this into words without sounding like a lovesick teenager, but the moment I saw him it was GAME OVER!

His arms around me. That little smile when he's trying not to look too relieved. My whole body was burning. Toe-curling, heart-skipping, I-definitely-still-love-you burning.

Then he kissed me.

Jesus. That kiss!

That FIRST kiss in what feels like for ever.

It was so intense I swear I forgot how to breathe.

And then, well ... I won't go into graphic details, but let's just say I'm exhausted. And it's not from trekking. My Fitbit clocked a heart rate of 189. It actually buzzed and asked if I was okay!

I don't know where we go from here. But I'll tell you one thing – there's no turning back!

Entry 39 – Post-Vietnam Reflections

I've been back for a few weeks now, so let's see how I'm getting on with that checklist:

> ✓ *Live a little. There's nothing wrong with a bit of drama. Bring on the chaos! – It's certainly been chaotic since we got back. But it's good chaos.*
>
> ✓ *Take holidays – Already booked a trip to Crete with Kev.*
>
> ✓ *Make time for friends who ask, "How are you?" and actually want to hear the answer – Dinner with Nico next month, and we see James and Richie at least three times a week. Also met up with Julie ... and her husband (!).*

✓ *Keep walking* – Trying my best ... but I must admit it's more difficult to get out of bed for those early-morning hikes these days.

✓ *Work no more than a forty-hour week* – Not quite, but Lorena's been a great help, so I'm down to fifty.

✓ *Take weekends off* – Well, Sundays, anyway.

✓ *Continue to support the charity* – I've started volunteering at Jersey Cheshire. I visit the residents every Wednesday evening for a chat and a cuppa. They've even asked if I'd like to join the board. How cool is that!

✓✓✓ *Find a man to love (or take a chance with one you've already found)* – No comment necessary

✓ *Don't hold grudges* – Getting there.

☐ *Stop trying to prove to Dad that you're good enough. He already knows I'm good enough. I just need to believe it myself* – Working on it.

✗ *Stop listening to Karen* – NO! I've realized she's an important part of me.

✓ *Tell James I'm Katie Green* – Told him on the summit. I think he was tempted to push me off!

And I guess that pretty much wraps up the great trek journal.

I'll need to start a new one. I suspect next year will be a big one.

Trek Training Progress Chart

Category	Status	Comments
Number of training walks	27½	That half walk counts. Don't argue.
Early wake-ups (5:15 a.m.)	11	Triggered by overthinking or Karen.
Poonamis	1	But that was enough!
New pairs of walking boots	3	Broken in and emotionally broken by.
Emails read and reread	25,561	Some educational, most alarming.
Blisters acquired	6	3 named: Abby, Clara, and Lily. Beautiful creatures.
Calories rationalized	All	"It's protein if it's in a flapjack, right?"
Times Karen was told to feck off	1,072	Including twice in the Co-op. Apologies to fellow customers.
Outfits coordinated to look like a professional mountain guide	9	Full Patagonia sponsorship pending.
Group walks survived	25	See also "New pairs of walking boots" and "Blisters acquired".

Category	Status	Comments
Times close to quitting	5	Exactly equivalent to the number of times snacks ran out.
Confidence level	Ranged from 1 to 11	Like a rollercoaster on espresso.
Emotional breakthroughs	Too many to count	Motto: "Just keep swimming." And if that fails: "Just keep swearing."

Donna Abel

Supporting

Jersey Cheshire Home

A Trek with Purpose. Throughout this story, you've followed one woman's messy, honest, and unexpected journey, one that began with a charity auction and led to something far greater than a physical trek. At the heart of it all was a cause that mattered deeply: **Jersey Cheshire Home**.

Who They Are

Jersey Cheshire Home is the only residential facility in Jersey dedicated to supporting people with complex physical disabilities. They provide not just care, but opportunity, dignity, and community — helping individuals live as independently and meaningfully as possible. They do this with genuine kindness, respect, and love.

Their team of dedicated professionals and volunteers offers 24-hour nursing care, physiotherapy, emotional support, and a safe, empowering environment tailored to each resident's unique needs.

Why It Matters

When you trek, sponsor, donate, or share their story, you help support:

- Residents, through no fault of their own, are living with conditions such as multiple sclerosis, motor neurone disease, strokes, brain injuries, and spinal injuries.
- Vital equipment and therapies that enhance mobility, communication, and independence.
- Programs that focus on living, not just surviving, art, music, outings, fitness, and more.

How You Can Help

Donate
Every contribution, big or small, makes a difference.
www.jerseycheshirehome.je/donate

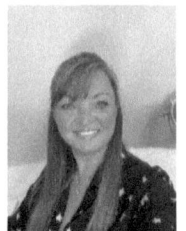

About the Author

Donna Abel brings heart, humour, and hard-earned wisdom to everything she does, be it trekking through remote landscapes or navigating boardrooms.

Donna is driven by purpose, compassion, and a desire to make a real difference. She writes with fierce wit, emotional depth, and the candour of a best friend sharing far too much over coffee.

Equal parts hilarious and heartfelt, *Lost and Found: The Misadventures of a Reluctant Trekker* is her first novella.

www.ingramcontent.com/pod-product-compliance
Lightning Source LLC
Chambersburg PA
CBHW020340010526
44119CB00048B/547